Back Pain

Michael Humphrey

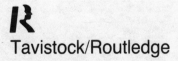

Tavistock/Routledge

First published in 1989 by
Routledge
11 New Fetter Lane, London EC4P 4EE

© 1989 Michael Humphrey

Phototypeset by Input Typesetting, London
Printed and bound in Great Britain by
Biddles Ltd, Guildford and King's Lynn

British Library Cataloguing in Publication Data

Humphrey, Michael
  Back pain.
  1. Man. Back. Backache
  I. Title II. Series
  616.7'3

ISBN 0–415–01720–3 hbk
ISBN 0–415–01721–1 pbk

Contents

Tables and figures

Acknowledgements

I am particularly grateful to Robin Bendall, Consultant Orthopaedic Surgeon at St George's Hospital, for his insistence on
valuing the role of the clinical psychologist in pain management.
I also thank Dr David Jenkins, Director of the Wolfson Medical
Rehabilitation Centre, for welcoming my modest contribution
there over the past twelve years.

Editorial guidance from Ray Fitzpatrick and Stan Newman has
improved the text, although they cannot be held entirely responsible for any residual blemishes. I am greatly indebted to Sue
Arnold and Karyna Gilvarry for allowing me to draw on their
word-processing skills without protest at my pedantry. Finally I
must record my appreciation of all that my patients have taught
and continue to teach me about the experience of pain.

Michael Humphrey
November 1988

Editors' preface

Clinical psychologists play an important and growing role in the provision of health care. Pain management is one area in which therapy based upon psychological principles is increasingly advocated. Back pain is an extremely common and often intractable problem. It may have an enormous impact on the individual sufferer's life and is responsible for considerable time lost from work. Both conventional and alternative medical therapies play a large role but with often limited efficacy. Back pain therefore poses a fundamental challenge to the psychologist in practice.

Michael Humphrey approaches this problem from the position of an experienced clinician who has worked for many years in a multidisciplinary back pain clinic. In this book he offers us the insights that this wide-ranging experience has provided. In a distinctively personal statement he uses excerpts from case reports to delineate the different dimensions of patients' experiences of back pain. He provides an accessible introduction to the diverse range of concepts and treatments currently being developed by clinical psychologists.

Chapter one

Medical aspects

Introduction

This book is one of a series commissioned to address the subjective
aspects of illness, and hence is written from a social and psychological rather than a medical standpoint. Nevertheless it seems
wise to begin with what is known about the medical aspects, if
only to set what follows in a sensible perspective. As a clinical
psychologist, I have worked closely with doctors from various
specialties for many years. These include the specialties principally
involved in the medical management of back pain, namely ortho-
paedics, rheumatology, neurology, and neurosurgery. Participating in a weekly clinic for patients with unsolved problems affecting
the lumbar spine (or mainly so) has meant exposure to all these
fields of expertise, and a few others besides.

Many of these patients have been referred for a first or second
opinion on the merits of surgery for the relief of pain, and some
are undoubtedly puzzled if not resentful at being confronted with
a psychologist. An explanation in terms of needing to look at the
owner of a bad back as well as the back itself is not always
received with good grace. Chronic pain patients are sensitive to
rejection and in constant fear of being discredited. After all, the
pain is real enough to them; and much more often than not, it
has already proved a major disruptive force in their lives. There
is no intention of trying to 'explain away' their disorder on a
psychological basis, yet equally it must be recognized that an
exclusively mechanical approach poses hazards of its own. The two
approaches should be seen as complementary, with the emphasis
shifting somewhat from case to case or even in the same case over
time.

Ideally a clinic of this nature calls for a psychologically sophisticated doctor as well as a psychologist with more than a layman's grasp of anatomy and physiology. Such partnerships are far from ubiquitous, and specialized attention to chronic back pain is unlikely ever to become the norm within the NHS. The St George's Hospital clinic owes much to the pioneering efforts of Waddell and his colleagues in Glasgow (Waddell *et al.* 1980; Waddell, Bircher *et al.*, 1984; Waddell, Main *et al.* 1984; Waddell 1987), who have given chapter and verse to the crucial distinction between disease and illness behaviour in the context of back pain. Like Wiltse and Rocchio (1975) earlier in the USA, they have underlined the value of a multidisciplinary team, which younger doctors exposed to the 'new look' in medical education are fast learning to appreciate. Far from negating the need for a series of monographs on the experience of illness, such healthy developments in the management of a commonplace yet extremely distressing disorder can only serve to highlight it.

Before turning to the structure of the vertebral column, and thence to the causes of back pain, two introductory statements can be made which have a bearing on pain in general and not merely on that emanating from the lumbar spine. First, it must not be forgotten that pain has an essentially biological purpose as nature's warning signal that all is not well with the organism. In certain circumstances an astute clinician will hesitate to prescribe pain-killing drugs for fear of masking a diagnosis that may point towards life-saving measures. The severe distress of an ectopic pregnancy is one of many examples that come to mind. The conscientious physician, especially when called upon to respond appropriately to all comers as in primary care, soon learns to look upon pain as a major ally in the fight against disease. He will be wary of the patient who cannot adequately communicate the experience of pain, or who is poor at localizing it. Individuals with the rare handicap of *congenital intensitivity to pain* (Baxter and Olszewski 1960; Sternbach 1963) are at a lifelong disadvantage in being unable to *feel* pain, so that various reflex responses – e.g. withdrawing the hand from a hot stove – are absent. Medical emergencies (such as ruptured appendix) may prove fatal through lack of the associated pain experience that is normally a guide to action. The rest of us are more fortunate in being able to develop the capacity for self-preservation. Even back pain, for all its generally benign character, is occasionally a sign of malignant disease calling for swift response and possibly heroic measures.

The second general statement is that many if not most episodes of pain are self-limiting. Even where there is a detectable underlying cause, the prospects for spontaneous remission are far from negligible. Medical intervention may help, yet for pain to disappear of its own accord is by no means unusual. This may be why warmth and bed rest have remained the first line of defence against acute back pain, regardless of its suspected origin. Studies from general practice have left no doubt that family doctors rely heavily on empirical treatment, and would be lost if this did not get the majority of their patients moving again. The question of prime interest to us is how and why some episodes of back pain, with an initial presentation that is in no way out of the ordinary, fail to remit within a matter of days or weeks. When the condition persists for several months, in the absence of any obvious remediable cause, the sufferer is well on the way to becoming 'chronic'. At what point it makes sense to categorize the patient in this fashion is debatable, but an earlier review of the literature (Humphrey 1980) revealed that six months was a commonly accepted milestone. To predict at the outset which patients are most at risk of sliding into long-term illness would be a valuable exercise, but at present we know all too little about the natural history of persistent back pain.[1] All that can be said with certainty is that chronic pain of any kind, whatever the causal factors, is not only devoid of any obvious biological purpose but is a major problem in its own right. Social and psychological aspects, whilst still poorly understood, will be reviewed as far as possible in later chapters.

Although we are still a long way from understanding why some individuals are so much more vulnerable than others to back pain, it seems reasonable to assume that more than one factor is involved. Meanwhile insight into the nature of pain mechanisms has been growing quite rapidly, especially in regard to the endorphins, those powerful pain-blocking chemicals that occur naturally in the brain and spinal cord. A recent review of the current status of back pain management by Wells (1985), on behalf of the Office of Health Economics, concluded that fundamental research of this kind might well hold the key to clinical progress. Be that as it may, an extended discussion of pain mechanisms would take us beyond the scope of this short book. For an informative guide to work in progress, the reader may wish to consult Melzack and Wall (1988).

The structure of the spine

The human spine comprises five basic components, namely bones, discs, ligaments, muscles, and nerves, together with a central space known as the spinal canal. Porter, in a brief but persuasive handbook for back pain sufferers, writes of a

> fascinating beauty of design about the spine, with its structure well suited for its complicated function. So often we hear that back pain is the result of poor anatomical design, that man's spine has not adapted to his upright posture. Not a bit of it. It is a miracle of design. . . . Problems arise when we expect too much, and abuse our backs. It is a wonder of engineering which we are only just beginning to investigate, and if respected it should serve us well without problems. Unfortunately, we tend to learn this too late when the damage has been done. Everything has a breaking point, however good the design, and if you apply too much stress,[2] it will fail. Do not blame the design.
>
> (Porter 1983: 6)

The twenty-four spinal bones, or vertebrae, are stacked rather like a tower of blocks, the lowest five (lumbar) vertebrae being most relevant to the transmission of backache. Each can move a little in relation to the adjacent one, so that the spine as a whole is rather like a flexible rod. Most of the load is taken by the vertebral bodies, those solid blocks of bone at the front; and each body is separated from its neighbour by a cartilaginous disc which acts as a shock-absorber. The vertebrae increase in size towards the base of the spine, the lowest being particularly strong in order to support the rest of the spine above it. Behind the vertebral body is an arch of bone with three projections, one at the back (the spinous process) and two at the side (the transverse processes). Muscles and ligaments are attached to these processes so that the spine can move freely without disintegrating. Two small joints (facet joints) are formed in the arch of bone behind the vertebral body to link up with similar joints at the next vertebra. The ring of bone formed by the arch of the vertebral body

Figure 1.1 : Structure of the spine (from the front)

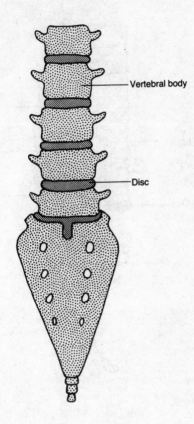

Vertebral body

Disc

Source: Porter 1983.

envelops the spinal canal, which varies in both shape and volume between individuals. This canal encloses the spinal cord in its upper part and a thick bundle of nerves in the lower part.

The structure, which may sound a bit complex as thus described, becomes easier to grasp with the help of the three-dimensional model of the lumbar spine familiar to anatomy students. It is to be hoped, however, that even two-dimensional illustrations will help to clarify the description (Figures 1.1 and 1.2).

Porter's handbook gives prominence to the displacement of an intervertebral disc as one of the commonest sources of back pain.

Figure 1.2 : Structure of the spine (from the side)

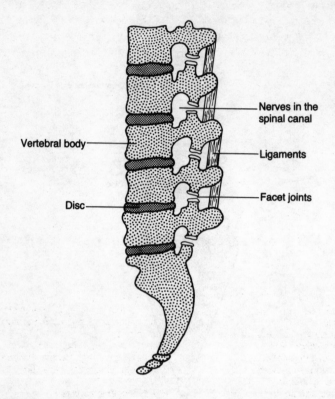

Nerves in the
spinal canal

Vertebral body

Ligaments

Facet joints

Disc

Source: Porter 1983.

Certainly it is far from rare, especially among the physically active, and it is not usually hard to diagnose. Overall, however, it accounts for only about 25 per cent of cases reaching medical attention (Wells 1985). Nerve root compression is a characteristic feature of 'slipped disc', giving rise to the unpleasant symptom of sciatica which can also occur in other circumstances. Here the pain radiates downwards via the sciatic nerve, sometimes as far as the feet, though it may not be all that easy to localize. The fact that a patient may specifically complain of sciatica is not much of an aid to the clinician, in that self-diagnosis has always been notoriously unreliable.

Aetiology of back pain

Although it may be entered as a diagnosis in clinical case notes, back pain is quite obviously a symptom rather than a disease. A broad classification of disorders known to trigger it is provided in Table 1.1, which is derived from another orthopaedic surgeon (Edgar 1984). Strictly medical causes, which include inflammatory conditions, metabolic disturbances, and neoplasms, are easily recognized as a rule, yet altogether they account for only a very small proportion of all cases of persistent backache (Jayson 1984).

Table 1.1 The causes of back pain

A. Mechanical and traumatic causes	*C. Neoplastic causes*
Musculotendinous and ligament strains	Primary benign tumours
	Primary malignant tumours
Fractures of the spine	Metastatic disease
Prolapsed intervertebral disc	
Spondylolysis and spondylolisthesis	*D. Metabolic bone disease*
Instability syndrome	Osteoporosis
Congenital anomalies	Osteomalacia
	Paget's disease
B. Inflammatory causes	
Discitis	*E. Referred pain*
Osteomyelitis	*Potential sources:*
Tuberculosis	Visceral, e.g. posterior duodenal ulcer
Brucellosis	Retroperitoneal, e.g. carcinoma of the pancreas
Paravertebral abscess	
Sero-negative B27 spondylarthropathies	Urinary tract, e.g. renal colic
Ankylosing spondylitis	Gynaecological, e.g. dysmenorrhoea
Reiter's syndrome	Pelvic, e.g. carcinoma of rectum
Psoriatic arthropathy	
Bowel associated	*F. Psychogenic causes*
Ulcerative colitis	*Pain associated with:*
Crohn's disease	Acute anxiety
	Depression

Source: Edgar 1984.

In much the same way, sensations of pain attributed to the back but actually originating elsewhere in the body can generally be elucidated from a careful history supplemented by special investigations. Psychogenic causes are probably the most controversial of those listed in the table. As Wood (1980: 6) has observed:

Too often this label reflects little more than a lack of detectable physical signs, and it scarcely identifies any underlying psychopathology to which treatment could be directed. Moreover, the concept carries with it the hazardous implication that no physical disorder is present and, conversely, that individuals with back pain due to obvious physical causes have no psychiatric or psychological problem.

It is worth repeating what has often been stated in other contexts, that no complaint appearing under a physical guise should be ascribed to psychological causes merely through exclusion of overt physical causes – on the contrary, there should always be positive grounds for entertaining an explanation in psychological terms. There is not much doubt that psychological factors can play a part – and sometimes a very large part – in maintaining an individual's pain experience, but it does not follow from this that they can give rise to it *de novo*. So while the exact cause of any particular episode may remain obscure, and there is some warrant for assigning back pain to the category of psychosomatic disorder, caution must be exercised in dismissing the idea of an essentially physical basis for the great majority of cases.

The orthopaedic influence emerges also in the common assumption that mechanical causes of back pain predominate. Would that all forms of it were as straightforward to diagnose as prolapsed intervertebral disc! Often enough the nature and origin of the mechanical defects assumed to be responsible for the pain remain shrouded in mystery. It is well known, for instance, that degenerative changes affecting bones and joints may be clearly revealed on standard X-rays without necessarily identifying the source of pain. In three surveys embracing a total of 1,702 persons, the difference between the proportion of those with and those without definite radiological evidence of degeneration of the lumbar discs who complained of low back pain was of no great magnitude: 59 per cent versus 47 per cent (Lawrence 1977). I recall with wry amusement how a medical colleague responded when I consulted her informally some years ago during an episode of partially incapacitating back pain. I was advised against undergoing an X-ray examination in case it might bring to light abnormalities of uncertain relevance! The advice was gladly accepted and the episode soon resolved without medical treatment.

Yet recent technical advances, such as *computerized tomography* (CT) and *magnetic resonance imaging* (MRI), have led to significant improvements in the diagnosis and management of mechanically determined back pain. The MRI scan in particular can show the quality of intervertebral discs in clear relief and also give useful information about nerve root compression. Such techniques have the undeniable merit of being non-invasive, unlike *discography*, which involves injecting a radio-opaque medium into the disc itself, a procedure every bit as unpleasant as it sounds. On the debit side they are costly, not yet widely available, and may temporarily mitigate the doctor's sense of therapeutic impotence at the expense of raising false hopes in the patient.

Myelography has for many years been the standard X-ray investigation used mainly to reveal evidence of nerve root compression by injecting a contrast medium into the spinal canal. Adverse reactions to this invasive procedure are said to have become rarer with the introduction of a water-soluble medium. It is used particularly by neurosurgeons, who are possibly more alert to the possibility of space-occupying lesions such as tumours and abscesses. Yet sciatic pain suggestive of nerve root entrapment may persist in spite of one or more negative myelograms, and the impact of such fruitless investigations upon the patient has yet to be systematically evaluated. It will be to the patient's advantage if myelography is superseded by the newer and non-invasive techniques mentioned in the previous paragraph, which are undoubtedly more efficient.

Traumatic causes of back pain have never loomed as large as mechanical causes, whether known or presumptive. Recovery from vertebral fracture is often surprisingly complete, with the associated pain unlikely to become chronic.[3]

The other main categories listed in Table 1.1 include a number of comparatively rare disorders associated with back pain, e.g. brucellosis, Reiter's syndrome, and Paget's disease. Some of the potential sources of referred pain are common enough, notably duodenal ulcer and dysmenorrhoea, but only a minority of sufferers from these conditions will complain of persistent and troublesome back pain. Primary tumours, be they malignant or benign, seldom develop in the spinal cord. In contrast, bony metastases are an all too familiar consequence of malignant tumours developing elsewhere in the body. Breast cancer is an outstanding example, with an incidence already above 5 per cent in women and believed to be on the increase. An insidious onset means that it may have started to spread before the primary tumour is discovered, and spinal metastases may well be perceived as a death sentence by patient and doctor alike. Even so, it is worth stressing that a history of breast cancer is most unusual among the women attending our weekly back pain clinic at St George's, many of whom have yet to reach the age of maximum risk. Thus although 'neoplastic causes' deserve to appear in a comprehensive catalogue, in practice the kind of back pain that forms the subject matter of this book is quite distinct from the pain of malignant disease.

In summary of this section, lumbar pain may arise from inflamed nerves, strained muscles or ligaments, or degenerative processes affecting bones and joints. More often than not the exact cause is speculative, with no clear evidence of injury in about 70 per cent of people who suffer from chronic back pain (Loeser 1980). However, in some 25 per cent of acute cases all the evidence may point to a slipped disc. Even the latter may prove to be self-correcting with complete rest but, as with other mechanical causes, the risk of recurrence is sufficient to create massive anxiety in some patients and a flourishing livelihood for some of the helping professions. And effective management becomes harder than ever when diagnostic ambiguity is compounded by individual reaction to the miseries of chronic or recurrent back pain. For, as with any other disorder that deserves to be taken seriously, what the patient wants and expects from the doctor is a concise explanation of how and why it has occurred and – more important still – a reassuring and convincing prognosis. Any clinician able to convey a confident grasp of past events without fear of contradiction by future events would be well on the way to making a fortune!

The size of the problem

It is now widely acknowledged that back pain is a symptom experienced by a large majority of the population at some time in their lives, at least 80 per cent according to the National Back Pain Association. By any standards it is a major cause of personal suffering and national economic loss. A former Minister of Health who was also a doctor (David Owen) was prompted to set up a multidisciplinary working group, whose recommendations were published a few years later (DHSS 1979). The social and industrial consequences of back pain have remained a matter of parliamentary interest to this day, yet there is, unhappily, little evidence of any improved understanding of the causes and remedies, or any reduction of the burden on the community over the past ten years.

In a study by Morrell and Wale (1976) of almost 200 women aged 20–44 who kept health diaries for four consecutive weeks, back pain was recorded as the third commonest symptom after headache and tiredness. More remarkable perhaps is the finding by Ingham and Miller (1979: Table 1) that as many as 21 per cent of a random sample of over 700 patients aged 16–75 who were registered with a Scottish health centre, but had not seen their GP for at least three months, reported at interview that they were suffering from back pain. Again, Dunnell and Cartwright (1972: Table 4) in their well-known study of resort to medication found that exactly the same proportion (21 per cent) of a nationwide stratified sample of more than 1,400 people on the electoral register had experienced backache during the fortnight preceding the interview. Whilst data of this kind cannot be used to derive a reliable estimate of the number of people in the nation at large who develop back pain in a specified period of time, they hint at a figure of awesome magnitude.

Fortunately for the medical profession, most of these episodes are brief and not severe enough to bring in a doctor. Dixon (1980), for example, has calculated that only 10 per cent of episodes reach medical attention. Nevertheless, on the basis of an earlier survey of morbidity in general practice (RCGP 1979) it has been estimated that 2.2 million individuals annually consult their GP on account of backache. This would mean that backache accounts for more than three times the morbidity attributable to coronary heart disease. So although rarely lethal in its effects upon the individual, it is extremely disruptive for society.

There is still no consistent picture of the action taken as a result of such consultations. In the often quoted general practice study by Dillane et al. (1966), 11 per cent of male but only 7 per cent of female patients were referred for specialist opinion on treatment, or a little over 9 per cent for the sexes combined. More recent estimates have been higher, with 12 per cent quoted by Glass (1979) and 17.5 per cent by Wood and Badley (1980). Differences in the definition of back pain as well as in styles of management are likely to have contributed to these discrepancies, but it seems reasonable to conclude that the overall referral rate would lie somewhere between 10 and 20 per cent.

When it comes to hospital admission, the statistics from

England, Wales, and Scotland indicate that in recent years back pain has created rather more demand than respiratory disorders such as bronchitis and emphysema. This may seem surprising in view of the heavy toll exacted by chest disease in the winter months, but the Office of Health Economics (Wells 1985) report puts the matter in perspective by suggesting that fewer than 3 per cent of patients consulting a family doctor for back pain in any given year will be taken into a hospital bed. Most of these patients are admitted for observation and bed rest, sometimes with traction, or for diagnostic procedures which cannot satisfactorily be performed on an out-patient basis.

Treatment

What can be done for the persistent sufferer, with or without the need for admission to hospital? There is certainly no lack of palliative measures, which include oral medication (analgesics, anti-inflammatory agents, and muscle relaxants); injections (e.g. epidural steroids or anaesthetics); physical intervention such as manipulation, massage, local heat application, and use of a corset; counter-stimulation (transcutaneous electrical nerve stimulation and acupuncture); and – usually as a last resort – surgery. But the treatment of back pain is apt to be dominated by individual convictions. In commenting on the apparent efficacy of unorthodox practitioners, Dixon (1987: xii) has written: 'Each therapist has his own theory, ranging from the plausible to those which can only be described as systematised delusions.'

In a review of fifty-nine therapeutic trials Deyo (1983) was unable to find compelling evidence to support the use of commonplace measures such as bed rest, traction, or wearing a corset. He was critical of the scientific basis of most studies, and drew attention to the need for blindness to treatment on the investigator's part as well as for better methods of measuring compliance and outcome. Such criticisms have become almost ritualistic among those who seek to question the status quo, and seldom make a significant impact. Moreover, inconclusive findings from a controlled trial (even when competently conducted) cannot be said to rule out the possibility of genuine benefit to the individual sufferer. Proper evaluation of therapies for low back pain, however commendable, is likely to remain elusive. The problem of spontaneous remission has already been mentioned, as has the study of Dillane *et al.* (1966) who found that 44 per cent of patients consulting a GP for back pain recovered within a week, whilst a mere 8 per cent were still complaining after two months. An equally tiresome complication is the 'placebo effect', which expresses the well-known truth that many patients respond well to a credible treatment administered by a caring therapist.

Spinal surgery has a limited place in the relief of pain, accounting for not more than an estimated 10,000 operations annually in England and Wales (Wells 1985). Nerve root compression from a displaced disc is the commonest indication, and here surgical intervention is sometimes unavoidable, as where bladder function or the use of the legs is compromised. Spinal fusion as a means of counteracting mechanical wear and tear is less frequently undertaken, and calls for particularly careful selection of patients if it is to produce measurable improvement in the quality of life (Hamblen 1980; Nelson 1987). The role of the surgeon in pain relief requires a more penetrating discussion than would be appropriate in this opening chapter, and we shall return to it later. At our weekly clinic at St George's we have seen all too many patients whose pain experience has been unaffected or even made worse by injudicious operations, occasionally repeated more than once. Where chronic pain is the outcome rather than the cause of a miserably frustrating life, it would be naïvely optimistic to look to the surgeon's knife for a remedy. The suggestion by Thomas *et al.* (1983) that surgery may produce better results when undertaken sooner rather than later is interesting, but their study needs to be replicated as it was based on a possibly atypical sample referred to a neurologist.

Outlook for the chronic sufferer: a grey area

Enough has been said to make it abundantly clear that back pain is not an explicit disease entity. To quote from Wood (1980: 23) again, it is a symptom 'with distinct manifestations in various locations from diverse causes in dissimilar individuals in different situations'. Apart from the notorious 'slipped disc', which is apt to be diagnosed in the absence of sufficient evidence, there is no unequivocal pathology or aetiology; and as already noted, structural abnormalities seen on X-ray examination are not easy to correlate with the clinical symptoms. Doubtless this ambiguity is part of the reason why it has been said to produce 'as much if not more discomfort in those treating the condition as in those suffering from it' (Silverman 1977). The level of complaint and degree of disability are liable to fluctuate unpredictably. Chronic and recurrent back pain victims tend to exasperate their doctors by failing to improve when all the clinical indications suggest that they should. Alternatively, they may gain dramatic even if only temporary relief from their symptoms by magical means such as hypnosis, acupuncture, or faith healing. Small wonder if this particular species of suffering humanity has been known to elicit a variety of adverse reactions from its medical attendants, ranging from polite dismay to downright scepticism.

Reverting to the question of what can be done for those who not only fail to respond rapidly to simple measures but go on to defy more elaborate procedures, an honest but uncompromising answer would be, not much. Psychological approaches will be reviewed in Chapter 5, but at this stage of our knowledge it would be rash to claim that they hold out as much hope as their practitioners would like to believe. At present only a minority of clinical psychologists are attracted to pain of any kind as a field of professional activity, and their therapeutic skills remain largely unproven. The extent to which patients who have not been helped by orthodox practitioners are finding relief from alternative or complementary medicine also remains uncertain. Few osteopaths or chiropractors are medically qualified, and increasingly they are being called upon to deal with intractable back pain. But whilst the initial response to treatment may be positive, we do not know how often their clients' faith is rewarded in the long term.

That doctors themselves have recently become more sympathetic to fringe medicine emerged from a survey of 86 GP trainees, of whom as many as 70 (81 per cent) wanted education in techniques such as acupuncture, homoeopathy, and manipulation; and in addition, 12 of the group had already sent patients to nonmedical practitioners (Reilly 1983). Patients' own attitudes have been investigated, albeit on a small scale, in two recent studies (Higham *et al.* 1983; Moore *et al.* 1985). Higham and her colleagues found that over a third of their 64 patients receiving treatment for back pain at a rheumatological out-patient clinic had consulted fringe practitioners, mainly osteopaths – an experience matched by my own. Moreover all but four patients had resorted to one or more self-prescribed remedies during their out-patient therapy. Of the 56 patients responding to a follow-up enquiry by Moore *et al.*, two out of five reported significant improvement over a period of eight weeks from the methods of alternative medicine. The time is now ripe for more systematic studies of its effectiveness.

The poor track record of existing therapies for chronic back pain prompts us to ask whether prevention might hold the key. Ideally one should always look towards prevention in such a situation, but grounds for optimism here are flimsy to say the least. People doing heavy manual work, housewives, and pregnant women are among those most clearly at risk; automation may take care of some of the more back-breaking toil as time goes on, and it is also on the cards that more and more women will come to opt out of household management and child-rearing. Even so, there will always be an inescapable residue of spine-grilling activities to be performed by vulnerable human beings rather than by robots. It would be salutary to record that in industry, where back pain is a major cause of absenteeism, great strides have been made towards prevention. Such is unhappily far from true, indeed DHSS figures show that the number of certified days of incapacity due to back trouble has increased by more than 20 per cent in Britain over the past few years. Taken in conjunction with the annual cost to the NHS, which the Office of Health Economics (Wells 1985) has estimated at £156 million, the current state of play is scarcely reassuring.

Three main strategies have been pursued in an attempt to reduce the incidence of back pain in the workplace: pre-employment screening, training in correct techniques of handling equipment (or people, in the case of nurses, firemen, and ambulance attendants), and the application of ergonomic principles to the design of recurrent tasks. Progress has been tantalizingly slow although there has been helpful discussion of some of the obstacles, for instance by Stubbs *et al.* (1983) in relation to nursing and by MacDonald (1984) and Simpson (1984) on a broader front. Medical screening of job applicants or trainees (e.g. for nursing) has been hampered by a failure to identify appropriate criteria – it is not necessarily the person of robust physique who is least at risk. Technical advice is of limited value unless the at-risk worker is able to follow it scrupulously and consistently even at times of maximum stress. As for the third strategy, there can be no doubt that improvements in the design of equipment and the layout of the working environment could make a substantial contribution to the avoidance of back injury, which is not to say that every factory could be rendered foolproof. As the OHE report states, progress in prevention 'might be seen to depend on the application of all three strategies described above in combinations specifically designed to satisfy the requirements of different occupational settings' (Wells 1985: 16). This is surely a fitting challenge for occupational medicine, with continued help from social and behavioural scientists. But to develop this theme further would be to encroach upon the material of the next chapter.

Chapter two

Who suffers?

According to Melzack and Wall (1988) and Bond (1984), low back pain is the commonest of all pains. No detailed evidence is offered in support of this statement, yet it is in tune with clinical experience. It is also borne out by published reports on the management of chronic pain, notably from the Mayo Clinic (Swanson *et al.* 1976; Swanson *et al.* 1979). Pain patients admitted to residential programmes for behaviour modification and retraining in activities of daily living are predominantly in this category. Facilities of this kind have become more prevalent in the USA over the past fifteen to twenty years, largely thanks to the pioneering efforts of psychologists such as Sternbach (1974) and Fordyce (1976). Methods of management will be discussed in Chapter 5; meanwhile it must suffice to note that much has been learnt about the nature of back pain from studies of the rehabilitation process.

If the lumbar spine is indeed the most vulnerable part of the human anatomy as a source of pain and ensuing disability, there must be a reason for this. In the opening chapter Porter (1983) was quoted as refusing to lay the blame on poor anatomical design. However, he was writing as an orthopaedic surgeon rather than as an expert on human behaviour. In terms of behavioural demand, recurrent daily activities call for a healthy and unimpaired lumbar spine. It is hard if not impossible to learn to compensate for poorly functioning joints and muscles in that region by cultivating alternative modes of performance. There is an all-embracing character about the movements controlled by that part of the body, whereas the effects of injuries to other parts (except for the brain itself) are more circumscribed. An example may be given from my own experience. At the time of writing I am plagued with an apparent inflammation of the left elbow joint, not so far presented for medical inspection in view of its apparently benign character. Such an affliction can be irritatingly persistent, especially in tennis players and the like; yet for most of us it requires only minor adaptations, and certainly not prolonged bed rest. Even so, one must learn to perform a variety of everyday tasks in a different manner if one is to protect the affected joint and give it a chance to recover. And although actual loss of a limb might appear to constitute a major disability for *anyone*, those who have watched an amputee sportsman in action will realize what can still be achieved minus an arm or even a leg.[1]

In contrast, where some or all of the lower vertebral joints are inflamed it is easy to imagine the havoc this is bound to create for anybody used to leading an active life. Apart from the discomforts of the resting state (in a fair proportion of cases at least), any slight incipient movement may give rise to a warning twinge; sudden or injudicious movements may produce a sharp stab of pain, with consequences ranging from brief disturbance to total incapacitation. And whilst the nature and cause of the inflammation may remain obscure after full investigation, what matters is that the reality of the handicap will be only too visible. For all the variety of individual reactions to chronic back pain, restrictions imposed at the acute stage are considerably more uniform. Moreover, despite scope for travesty (as when an actor is required to portray a man in agony), downright malingering is rare in both my own and other writers' experience.

What is there to say about the kind of people who succumb to chronic low back pain? Granted that anyone ambulant is at risk of an acute or subacute episode, and probably more than once in a lifetime, how are we to recognize those who may be less than ordinarily adept at emerging from such an experience without ill effects? Further research is needed to identify those peculiarly at risk; meanwhile it may be helpful at this point to summarize what is known or believed about the characteristics of long-term sufferers.

Personal and social attributes

Most published studies have the disadvantage of being purely descriptive and devoid of acceptable control data. For example, it can serve no useful purpose to estimate the proportion of back pain sufferers even in a representative sample who are poorly educated or unhappily married (say) unless one has reason to believe that victims of other disorders – or indeed people not obviously handicapped in any way at all – are significantly different in these respects. It is well known that superior education goes with more effective use of medical and social resources, and to that extent is conducive to better health. The significance of other demographic factors is more debatable, but it is possible to glean a few useful hints from the literature where the findings from diverse studies are both reasonably consistent and broadly in line with clinical experience.

That chronic back pain sufferers are typically manual workers with a limited formal education has emerged from numerous studies over the past twenty years or more (e.g. White 1966; Beals and Hickman 1972; Nagi *et al.* 1973; Maruta *et al.* 1976). The findings of Nagi and his colleagues are especially likely to be replicated, in North America at least, because they were based on an epidemiological survey of well over a thousand persons aged 18–64 in Ohio, of whom more than one in six reported that they were often troubled by pain in the back. An inverse relationship was found between level of education and frequency of complaint; manual workers were in a majority and, somewhat unexpectedly, women outnumbered men in all occupational categories (21 per cent versus 14 per cent). The authors controlled for menstrual disturbance by showing that the sex difference held good beyond the age of 50, and they explained it at least partly in terms of the well-known discrepancies between male and female pain thresholds and anxiety levels. In so far as severity of complaint is the main determining factor in referral to a specialist, rather than the degree of observable (let alone measurable) dysfunction, we would expect women to present themselves more often even if they were not constitutionally more prone to the disorder in question. This is bound up with their greater use of the health services in general, which takes account of their greater readiness and freedom to visit doctors (see the General Household Survey published annually by the Office of Population Census and Surveys). The tendency of epidemiologists to rely heavily on self-report, if only as a matter of convenience, would also help to explain the apparently greater sufferings of female workers interviewed by Nagi *et al.* (1973). It would be wrong to attach too much weight to this discrepancy, which has not usually been reported by clinicians or research workers employing other methods to assess severity of pain or the need for specialized rehabilitation.

Clinical studies offer a less satisfactory basis for generalization, but a study by Gentry *et al*. (1974) yielded an intriguing perspective. Of fifty-six patients, two out of three were in 'hard manual or routinised clerical jobs', and almost one in five was a housewife. Tempting as it may be to focus on physical stress, this was seen as not necessarily the main factor. As the authors observe, many of their patients

> had experienced unmet dependency needs early in life. That is, they had begun work at an early age and had worked at relatively hard jobs for a long time prior to symptom onset. In addition, they were typically later-born children from large families, who in turn married early and quickly had several children of their own. Thus, by virtue of providing for others and not being able to fully depend on their own parents as children, they had postponed gratification of such needs until a minor injury provided a rational and socially acceptable means of depending on others for social and economic support.
>
> (Gentry *et al*. 1974: 176)

Some women seen at our weekly clinic have given such a history, albeit not often either strikingly or spontaneously. It was also elicited from a substantial minority of a group of patients attending the Wolfson Medical Rehabilitation Centre at Wimbledon (part of the St George's group) in the late 1970s. Thus 15 out of 39 married patients had three or more children, and all but four of this subgroup came from sibships of three or more (Humphrey and Jenkins 1982). The quality of the patient's family experience – marital and parental – is sometimes of overriding importance, or so it would appear. Convincing evidence from larger and less biased samples is still awaited, however. This aspect will be discussed further in Chapter 3.

It has long been known that consultations for back trouble reach a peak in the sixth decade and decline thereafter. Initial episodes would be expected to occur a good deal earlier in life, and indeed it must be comparatively rare for an individual to see a doctor on this account for the first time after the age of 50. Accidents affecting the spine can of course occur at any time, although here again the caution that will sooner or later replace the impetuosity of youth can be relied upon to exert a protective influence. Workers in the building trade, for instance, have been found to suffer more back injuries before the age of 30 than after that age, although older workers have longer periods of sick leave after comparable accidents (Stubbs and Nicholson 1979). In addition, the individual's overall lifestyle (including choice of leisure pursuits) will have a bearing on the hazards incurred. Sporting and other vigorous activities are bound to add to the risk of injury, and to make adaptation that much harder after it has occurred.[2]

Compared with age, sex, and occupation, marital status is a more controversial factor. Nagi *et al.* (1973) conceded that the relative immunity of never-married persons and the greater vulnerability of the widowed in their sample could have been largely due to the age factor, but they were alive to the possibility of a causal link in bereaved persons through the effect of inadequate social support on coping behaviour. An earlier study (Nagi *et al.* 1965) had produced evidence that back sufferers with a history of divorce, separation, or bereavement responded less well to a rehabilitation programme than married persons without such a history.

Bernard (1976) among others has argued that in some respects marriage confers more protection on men than on women, especially so far as psychiatric and psychosomatic disorders are concerned. Be that as it may, the implications of chronic pain are undoubtedly different for the two sexes, as will be made explicit in due course. Marital discord might well be more relevant to the persistence of handicap than marital disruption to which some will have had time to accommodate. Kreitman *et al.* (1965) drew attention to the possible bearing of unresolved marital problems on bodily complaints with no detectable organic basis. It has even been alleged that marital counselling can be successful in the relief of backache where more direct approaches have failed (Silverman 1977).

The influence of the family is further acclaimed by the above-mentioned study of Gentry *et al.* (1974). More than half of their patients reported one or more family members (parent, grandparent, sibling) as suffering from either low back pain or some other equally debilitating physical disorder such as arthritis, diabetes, or cancer. In addition, one patient in four made mention of 'significant others' with a history of chronic back trouble which had also failed to respond to conventional therapy. The absence of a control group is an obstacle to interpretation, yet the impact of family models on pain and illness behaviour has been evident for some time (e.g. Craig 1978) and confirmed by more recent studies (e.g. Violon and Giurgea 1984; Edwards *et al.* 1985). It is not hard to appreciate how growing up in an atmosphere of hypochondriacal self-concern amongst influential figures might predispose an individual towards escaping into invalidism when under stress; conversely, an attitude of stoicism in the face of discomfort could be inculcated and heavily reinforced within the family. Such considerations may apply particularly to back pain on account of its conspicuous and at times dramatic manifestations.

To summarize what has already been stated about the general characteristics of back pain sufferers: they are quite likely to be young if the pain has followed closely on a definite spinal injury, otherwise they are more likely to be middle-aged, especially where the condition has become chronic. It is less clear whether men or women are more at risk, since the heavier stresses borne by male manual workers may be counterbalanced by specific female stresses such as pregnancy, childbirth, and infant care (to say nothing of ordinary household tasks). The effect of occupational hazards upon the spine is a complex and controversial area, well reviewed by Anderson (1987), but there can be no real doubt as to the relevance of the workplace. Marital status as such is less sensitive as an indicator of vulnerability, in that it is compatible with a wide variety of lifestyles. Let us now go on to consider more specific categories of complainant.

Those who complain

The grievously injured

As stated in the opening chapter, there is no known history of injury in the majority of cases. Our own experience over the past few years of running a special clinic for chronic back pain sufferers has amply confirmed this statement. On the other hand a small minority of patients – probably not more than 5 per cent – have been injured so severely that they can be considered lucky to have survived. Such an event does not preclude the possibility of important psychological factors, which indeed may sometimes have contributed to a serious accident. The concept of the 'accident-prone personality' is oversimplified, yet there can be no doubt that some of us live more recklessly than others. Dangerous driving if practised for long enough will sooner or later result in an accident, and it may then be a matter of chance whether the driver and any passengers are injured, and if so how badly. Even when a person's injuries arise from another's recklessness, in the absence of any known predisposition towards accidents, the risk of adverse psychological consequences may be acute. And so the need for psychological evaluation in such cases remains. However, the physical aspects are likely to predominate more often than not, as may be sufficiently obvious even to the casual observer.

Examples from our series include a man who fell down a lift shaft, another who was catapulted violently against the side of a ship when aquaplaning in Poole harbour, and a woman who as a teenager had been thrown from a car that went out of control, and who over the years had made a miraculous recovery from tetraplegia. Probably the most gruesome accident had befallen a man who had always wanted to own a garage, and shortly after fulfilling this ambition had been crushed beneath a faulty hydraulic ramp when working on a car. Patients with this kind of history display their physical problems only too clearly, so that it does not require a clinical examination to establish that they are genuinely disabled. The spine may have become distorted, gait may be grossly abnormal, and usually there are neurological signs (which are rare among those who have not been grievously injured). As expected, the extent of recovery is variable, but rarely if ever has an ambulance been needed to bring them to the clinic.[3]

The ill-fated

We have seen a number of patients whose life has taken a sudden downward plunge, with ensuing loss of equilibrium and enhanced susceptibility to stress. The interval between key event and onset of pain varies widely, and in most cases it would be hazardous to infer a direct causal link. What stands out clearly in such patients is their reduced capacity for coping with life, especially where social support is inadequate. Studies of life events in relation to chronic pain have been conspicuous by their rarity; apart from a preliminary study by Rose (1975), who found an excess of signifi-cant events in back patients as compared with matched controls during the three months prior to consulting their GP, and a similar comparison by Feuerstein *et al*. (1985) which suggested that family stress had more adverse effects than pressure of work, there have been few useful leads in the literature. Yet *a priori* there would seem to be a case for anticipating a causal relationship of some kind.

A recent example of earlier misfortune is the woman of 55 referred from an orthopaedic hospital. The surgeon asked for help in solving a diagnostic puzzle arising from the all too familiar situation of persistent pain in the absence of positive findings. She was a simple soul, and her story was that at 19 she had married a man who was a few years older than herself. The marriage had worked well until mental illness supervened after about fifteen years. Without much warning her husband had become violent towards her and their two pre-adolescent children, so that she was fearful for their safety, to say nothing of her own. The police were called and he was compulsorily admitted to hospital. He refused to co-operate over the medication that might well have controlled his schizophrenic illness, and she was compelled to divorce him. Four years later he died of cancer, but she remained unable to create a new life for herself. Her sons had married and continue to live locally, but essentially she was all alone in the world. Her pain had developed a year or two before referral to the clinic, and recently her 78-year-old mother had been pressed into service as a home-help-cum-gardener whilst she herself led the life of a semi-invalid.

Illustrations within this broad spectrum of patients suffering as a result of recent life events could be multiplied. The historical detail is infinitely varied, but what most of these patients have in common is a readiness to throw in the towel despite strong protestations to the contrary. A history of an accident at work will usually mean an unresolved compensation claim; and some of these patients have been through an undeniably traumatic experience, like the young female who caught her hair in a machine and felt as though she had been scalped, or the ageing male who had a contretemps with a crane. Others might justifiably be accused of overdramatizing, but this is not the place to speculate upon their reasons for so doing. Not all authorities are agreed that there is such a thing as a 'compensation neurosis', and rapid resolution of the pain problem is by no means guaranteed to follow settlement of the claim.

It is not suggested that chronic pain comes as an inevitable sequel to the cruel stroke of fate, rather that the latter increases the patient's vulnerability and thus opens the way to a malignant chain of events. Given ordinary luck, if not a trouble-free life, he or she might never have experienced a pain problem; or if a painful episode had nevertheless occurred, it would most probably have run its course in the normal manner.

The surgical disaster

In a survey of 100 patients referred to me by an orthopaedic surgeon, 31 had a history of spinal surgery for the relief of pain (Humphrey and Jones 1987). At the time of writing three such cases (two men and a woman) were seen consecutively in the previous week, and by way of illustration it may be helpful to recapture some of the details.

A woman of 39 was referred by her general practitioner for a second orthopaedic opinion. The pain had first developed in her mid-20s, but she was not in severe discomfort at the time of her marriage to a naval officer at the age of 28. However, although the relationship has so far proved happy enough in terms of affection and companionship, married life has done nothing to improve the state of her back. In 1979, some eighteen months after her wedding, she underwent a laminectomy. This set the stage for a decline in the couple's sexual activity, but she was able to work full-time in support of her husband after he left the Navy to train as an accountant. But her pain persisted, and after two further operations in 1984 and 1985 she was obliged to hand over many domestic tasks to him and ultimately to give up her high-grade secretarial post. At the time of the psychological assessment she had resumed major responsibility for the home, yet was barely able to manage even two hours a week of voluntary work, which entailed reorganizing a filing system. Her pain had meanwhile shifted to the coccyx and was of variable intensity.

She had grown up in a secure middle-class home, but soon after leaving school she had nursed her mother through a distressing terminal illness. Thereafter her menstrual periods had ceased for ten years, returning only after six months of marriage. Anorexia nervosa had been suspected but never confirmed, and instead she had been diagnosed as suffering from glandular fever. It was in this setting that her back pain had later evolved; and while she had tended to favour sport at the expense of academic work at her small private school, she was forced to give up tennis and other vigorous pursuits. Before marriage she had made the most of her limited educational qualifications by working her way up from straight secretarial work to a more responsible position in the public sector; after marriage she had lived abroad for a while, which restricted her scope for outside work. Although she had always wanted children she had never really been in a position to pursue this aim consistently or wholeheartedly, and was now faced with the prospect of reconciling herself to a childless future.

She had sought help from a psychotherapist in the hope of improving her self-image, since with neither children nor career she had developed a sense of inadequacy tinged with resentment. The therapist had offered to see her regularly over the next few months, and meanwhile the couple were given detailed advice by the present writer on how to improve their sexual relationship. They were encouraged to report progress to me by telephone until their follow-up appointment at the back pain clinic, but failed to do so.

This story is unusual in several respects, notably as regards the complex medical history of which full details have not been given. An outstanding aspect is the failure of doctors to explore her psychological problems in relation to her back pain, but this is commonplace. After all, surgeons are not trained to investigate the owner of a bad back except from their own specialized stand-point, and would hesitate to refer on in the absence of a psychiatric history or overt psychological disturbance. Such patients com-monly present themselves with great conviction in their search for a physical solution to what they see as a physical problem, and they may move from one practitioner to another in growing desperation (though as it happens this woman had remained loyal to her original surgeon). Their satisfaction with key roles – occu-pational, social, marital – takes a downward plunge over the years, until it may become almost too late to rescue them from total despair.

The two men with histories of unsuccessful surgery had been handicapped for a shorter period.

The first of these was a self-employed architect aged 40, tall and courteous with a typical public school persona. He lived some way outside London but worked there during the week, so that he was able to attend the Wolfson Medical Rehabilitation Centre in the hope of overcoming the worst of his problems. He described his lumbar pain as having a special quality of its own, no longer acute but worse than a dull ache, and he was doubtful of being able to maintain his professional standards unless he could be relieved of it. He had worked mainly abroad from choice, and would have liked to resume this way of life. His wife was career-minded and there were no children.

Two years earlier he had undergone his first spinal operation, supposedly a laminectomy, which he regarded as 'more like an assault than surgery'. That said, he was not entirely unforgiving towards the orthopaedic surgeon, yet it may be significant that he consulted a neurosurgeon the following year about the possibility of a further operation to rectify the damage. This was duly performed, but it could not be determined exactly what had been done on the previous occasion. The second operation led to some relief from the associated sciatica but virtually none from the back pain. His latest contract had begun to make heavy demands upon him, and he was compelled to give up his principal recreations of golf and sailing. Sexual intercourse became difficult, although there was no suggestion of marital problems. His response to the rehabilitation programme was reported as somewhat tense, and this was borne out on a self-report questionnaire designed to measure anxiety both as a personality trait and as a current state of mind (Spielberger et al. 1970). When last seen a few months later he was holding his own, but his pain was largely unrelieved.

Here, then, was another unhappy story of chronic pain which surgery had left untouched. The marriage was of similar duration, and again there were no children, which may have been partly by design. There was perhaps a cumulative sense of disillusionment, but a degree of natural reticence made it hard for him to express the full extent of his anguish. It might have been helpful to interview his wife but there was no opportunity for this. As in the previous case, there was no record of any prior attempt to explore the meaning of the chronic pain for the individual.

The second man was also aged 40, but presented quite differently. Where the other two patients had acted normally enough during a leisurely interview, without much visible sign of pain, this patient displayed unmistakable signs of 'pain behaviour' albeit not to a gross extent. Similarly, his profile on the Minnesota Multiphasic Personality Inventory (MMPI) was of a kind traditionally associated with enhancement of pain experience by psychological factors (see Humphrey 1980). His laminectomy had been performed at least three years earlier.

This man had left school at 15 and, after starting an apprenticeship, had joined the Army in order to please his father to whom he had always been closely attached. Some years later he had sustained a leg injury, and it was whilst undergoing rehabilitation that he met his wife. He was subsequently invalided out, and married her when they were both 24. Some years before meeting him she had been severely injured in a car crash, but she was remarkably independent in view of the gravity of her handicap (she was paraplegic). She had a child by a previous marriage which had ended in divorce, and went on to have four more children by her second husband although the first of these died soon after birth. At the time of interview she was convinced that she was pregnant yet again, despite having been sterilized after her fifth child. The couple seemed more amused than worried about this, and were inclined to make light of their reduced circumstances (he had been off work for nine months, she was no longer earning). There could be little doubt that they were sustained by their religious faith as well as by their deep mutual commitment.

After his Army service he had joined the police force. It was while intervening in an assault during New Year revels that he had strained his back, and the onset of the pain was so acute that he thought he had been stabbed. He lay helpless on the ground until he could be taken by a police car to the nearest hospital, where he remained under observation for some while. Later he developed right-sided sciatica, which was relieved by the operation. He was not much better off, however, as it did not take long for the pain to return in his left leg. This was slow to improve, and he was off work for more than a year. On resumption he was switched to a desk job which he enjoyed, but the back and leg pain kept recurring. He estimated that he had worked for only six months all told during the three years preceding the interview, and his future was therefore uncertain.

For reasons that were not entirely clear he had fallen out with his surgeon at the other hospital, but he indicated that he would be willing to entrust himself to my orthopaedic colleague when we first saw him together. Although X-rays and CT scan showed clear evidence of degenerative changes in the lowest two intervertebral joints, a decision on management was postponed pending further investigations. The psychological assessment argued the need for caution, and the dynamics of his life situation might well repay further scrutiny.

It is almost superfluous to add that no attention had been paid to psychological aspects during the time that this tale of woe was unfolding. Hamblen (1980) has dismissed the need for routine psychological screening prior to spinal surgery for the relief of pain, and it could well be impracticable within existing constraints. He does, however, regard this as an essential precaution before repeat surgery, and one would like to hope that such a policy is gaining ground in Britain as well as in the USA. Objectively the unimproved patient may be no worse off, but when unrealistic expectations are confounded then lack of improvement may lead to subjective decline as well as keen disappointment. At the risk of succumbing to the complacency of hindsight, one cannot over-stress the folly of operating on a painful back without due regard for the personality and social circumstances of its owner.

The need for reappraisal

These few illustrations were intended to give some idea of the range of settings in which chronic low back pain has been found to evolve. Not every story is as complex or as dramatic as those selected from our case histories, but there is really no substitute for careful enquiry. This is part of the reason why back pain is on the whole rather poorly managed in the NHS, and not always much better in the private sector. A typical out-patient clinic leaves the busy surgeon short of time, and once the decision to operate has been taken events have a nasty habit of rolling on in a preordained sequence. The post-operative period after a laminectomy may be relatively uneventful, though it is more protracted after a fusion which usually entails several months' convalescence before return to work. Complications may develop as with any other form of surgery but fortunately they seem to be rare. It is when the hapless patient tries to pick up the threads of normal living again that trouble may be in store.

Spinal fusion is an elective operation, except possibly when undertaken as a palliative measure for metastatic cancer (which need not concern us here). The nature of the decision should be explained clearly to the patient, who should not be allowed to think of it as conferring a licence to punish his or her back as shamelessly as may have happened in the past. Laminectomy is also elective in the majority of cases, but may be performed as an emergency procedure either to restore bladder function or to obviate the risk of paraplegia from permanent damage to the nerves. Again care should be taken to protect the patient from false expectations, and it is not always made clear that disappearance of sciatica can be anticipated more confidently than total relief from back pain. Resumption of normal activities has to be planned, and there may be a need for specialized rehabilitation in some cases. Much will depend on the discrepancy between past and present lifestyles, and on future commitments. Here the heavy manual worker and the mother of pre-school children are equally at a disadvantage.

Of course not all back pain sufferers are surgical candidates, even at our own specialized clinic, nor are orthopaedic surgeons exclusively concerned with their management. However, the assumed prevalence of mechanical causes does mean that the orthopaedic clinic is often the first port of call when a specialist opinion is wanted. Indeed, it has been estimated that 25 per cent of patients attending such a clinic present with spinal problems of one sort or another (Dixon 1980). A further bias stems from my close collaboration with an orthopaedic colleague, but it must be remembered that back patients experience a variety of different management styles. Probably the main unifying factor is the medical practitioner's cursory interest in the patient as a person, but this continues to apply – with a few notable exceptions – to medicine as a whole.

What needs to be appreciated above all else is the profundity of the changes that may envelop the life of a chronic back pain sufferer within quite a short space of time. Different aspects of these changes will be considered more fully in later chapters, and here brief comment must suffice.

Schizophrenia, in many ways the deadliest of all mental afflictions, has been mentioned in passing; and readers with first-hand experience of the illness (or family of illnesses) will need no reminding that among chronic patients a life of dedicated idleness can rapidly become the norm, for soon all motivation to engage in purposeful activity is lost. Back pain sufferers do not experience the debilitating onslaught of psychotic thought disorder, yet once they have lost heart they may find themselves similarly cut off from society. Life begins to pass them by, with adverse effects on their self-reliance and self-esteem. Sooner or later they will be assailed by all the psychological problems of unemployment, they will become alienated from their loved ones, and depression will come to dominate their view of the world. In extreme cases suicidal thinking may take over, and already one of our own patients has put an end to her life, leaving a devoted husband and five grown-up children. Whereas actual suicide as an outcome of chronic pain may be rare, a growing sense of desperation is certainly not. There may be some healthy people who do not subscribe to the philosophy of that eccentric recluse, Henri Thoreau (1854), who wrote that 'the mass of men lead lives of quiet desperation'. But he had chosen to isolate himself in his self-made shanty in the woods of Massachusetts, which is a very different matter from being driven into the life of a hermit by chronic pain.

Chapter three

Marriage and family life

An area of growing interest in the management of chronic pain, but one where there is very little hard evidence on which to draw, is the patient's intimate relationships. Marriage affords an almost unique context wherein to explore the impact of pain experience and behaviour on daily life. Nowhere else is there opportunity for close encounters over such a prolonged period, with so much variation in the quality and stability of personal and social roles for each partner. And few other relationships between individuals provide the same scope for self-disclosure, or for acting and reacting against the stresses of daily life. Yet it is an essentially private experience, more amenable to the skills of the novelist than those of the social or behavioural scientist. 'People behind their hidden married screens have personalities quite different from those they usually reveal to their relatives, friends and acquaintances. Perhaps, in order to know a person really well, you have to marry them' (Beyfus 1968: xi).

Although hard evidence is scanty, it would appear that only a minority of chronic pain patients are unattached. For example, some 80 per cent of patients seen at our weekly back pain clinic are currently married, and most of the other 20 per cent have been married at some stage. This is not too surprising in view of the age distribution, with the majority in their 40s or 50s. What is perhaps more worthy of remark is the significantly greater proportion of never-married patients attending an orthopaedic clinic at the same hospital with minor complaints, and no history of chronic pain (Humphrey and Jones 1987). The two series of one hundred patients were carefully matched for age and sex, and turned out to be socially similar. Of the control group only two-thirds were married at the time of initial presentation, whilst almost half of the others had so far remained single. This finding, while unexpected, is in line with an earlier report on a more miscellaneous series of pain patients (Merskey and Spear 1967). The potential destructiveness of chronic pain and disability, in a relationship where the other partner is usually active and pain-free, requires no emphasis. The paradox of enhanced marital stability among pain patients (if such it is) has only recently begun to attract attention, and its interpretation has been discussed in a preliminary study of psychogenic pain (Hughes *et al.* 1987). We shall return to it later, but it might be instructive at this point to recall some arresting comments from a distinguished neuro-surgeon which were widely reported at the time of his presidential address to the Neurology Section of the Royal Society of Medicine. He wrote as follows (Connolly 1982: 162):

> A great hazard to women is painful neurosis induced by a 'golden husband'. He listens assiduously to all her symptoms, carefully notes them, remembers each day to enquire about them in detail, and when she visits the doctor he fills in the minutiae which she has failed to relate. He cultivates neurosis, and any lady feeling that her husband sometimes tends to be a little neglectful and brusque should be grateful that he is not over-attentive and sympathetic, for when leucotomy for depression was much in vogue, many of the women patients proved to be suffering from 'golden husbands'.

Connolly does not explain why he singled out the male partner for these sharp comments, which may equally apply to the female partner. Perhaps it relates in some way to conventional expectations of male and female roles in marriage.

The partner's attitude

The fact that many painful conditions tend towards a peak incidence in middle life has advantages for the clinician who is prepared to look beyond the identified patient. If marriage or some other form of stable partnership is normal at this stage, it will ideally provide not only an extra source of information but also a potential therapeutic ally. We have long made a practice of interviewing the partner whenever possible at our weekly clinic, and there have been occasions when his or her elusiveness has turned out to be a signal that all was not well with the relationship. But as already hinted, overt marital problems are exceptional among our clientele. Rather, we have learnt to be on the lookout for a collusive element, which may range from the crassly conspicuous to the carefully camouflaged. Quite clearly this kind of interplay is not to be regarded as pathological in itself, and indeed some measure of complementarity is needed for a marriage to survive – why else should a couple elect to remain together unless they are capable of at least partially fulfilling one another's emotional needs? It is only where the partner's collusive behaviour has gone beyond all sensible bounds, and usually over a long period, that trouble may set in.

Before discussing the harmful effects of marital collusion it may be helpful to recall a case where the husband's caring attitude towards his pain-ridden wife had apparently always been a positive factor in their marriage.

When seen in mid-1985 the couple had been married for more than 20 years, having known each other for only a few months before the onset of her back trouble during rope-swinging exercises when she was a physical education student. He was an only child who had helped his mother to look after his sick father from an early age until his teenage years, when the father died. Thus he embarked on marriage with a realistic concept of what illness can do to family life, and later gave up a more lucrative career in the services for a teaching post in a local school at least partly in order that he could attend to her needs more effectively. During the past four years she had undergone two spinal operations which had failed to rescue her from a state of semi-invalidism, although she had recovered well from a previous hysterectomy. The family lived about a hundred miles from London, but the patient was referred to St George's Hospital by her local rheumatologist at the age of 44 for an opinion on the wisdom of further surgery.

After psychological assessment I wrote as follows to my orthopaedic colleague: 'I am sure that this couple totally live for one another despite the devastating effects of the chronic pain problem, to which the two children have learnt to accommodate over the years. Like you I am convinced that the problem is basically a mechanical one, and the tendency towards depression is in no way a contraindication to further surgery.' Some nine months later she underwent a third spinal fusion, and when seen briefly before her discharge from hospital it was almost as if she had simultaneously undergone a personality transformation. Another 15 months after this the couple were seen at home on a social visit, mainly with a view to enlisting their co-operation in vetting parts of this book. She was obviously in fine fettle, and had recently taken steps towards resuming part-time work of a non-strenuous nature.

Here the wife's disability had at times virtually immobilized her, and the couple's social life was grossly restricted. Holidays were a thing of the past, although the husband had bought a motor caravan in the hope of making good this deficiency. But whereas overall the disruptive effects of chronic pain were no less than in many other cases seen over the years, an exceptional feature of this case was the husband's realistic understanding of his role. The impression conveyed on the home visit was that he had no compelling need of his own to suffocate her, any more than she had an overwhelming need to control or exploit him. A Marital Patterns Test (Ryle 1966) given at the initial interview yielded evidence of a healthy exchange of affection in the context of an egalitarian relationship. Interestingly, at their own suggestion the patient's GP had referred her to a psychiatrist some years earlier, whose verdict after a couple of sessions was that the problem was essentially physical.

The need for extra caution in deciding on a second (let alone a third) spinal operation for the relief of pain, as advocated by Hamblen (1980), is nevertheless borne out by this story. Surgical fools rush in where psychological angels fear to tread, but fortunately there are growing indications that the era of the knife-happy surgeon is on the way out. As always, there is an element of luck in the outcome of these recurring dilemmas, and one can hardly expect to get it right every time. What must be avoided at all costs is recourse to surgery as a means of resolving personal or marital problems. That will never work.

The influence of an over-protective spouse in holding up recovery from serious illness or disablement has been noted in other contexts, even if the evidence is largely anecdotal. More compelling is the evidence from a study by Block *et al.* (1980), who demonstrated that patients would rate their pain as more severe in the presence of a solicitous spouse as compared with a neutral observer (ward clerk), whereas the opposite applied to patients with a non-solicitous spouse. Moreover the well-supported group had a significantly longer history of pain complaint (mean 15.5 years) than the poorly supported group (mean 4.5 years), which suggests that unhealthy reinforcement may have occurred at least to some extent. Indeed, the authors offered two possible explanations for their intergroup difference. The first was that patients might be more likely to develop chronic problems when pain behaviour was heavily and consistently reinforced by the partner, as predicted by the operant model. The second possibility was that the quality of the partner's response might be open to some form of natural selection in the course of chronic disability:

> During the first few years of illness some spouses may respond to pain behaviour with anger or frustration but, with increasing chronicity, many spouses may either adapt to the situation and respond to pain displays in a reinforcing manner, or leave the marriage.
>
> (Block *et al*. 1980: 251)

In so far as the nature of marital interaction is likely to fluctuate over time, and may be far from constant even for short periods, it seems reasonable to suggest that these two explanations are not mutually exclusive.

An ingenious experiment by Block (1981) took the argument a stage further. Spouses of chronic pain patients were asked to rate videotapes of both neutral and painful facial expressions emitted by their partners, as well as by hospitalized chronic pain patients and healthy volunteers, while their physiological reactions were monitored. Increased galvanic skin response and (to a lesser extent) heart rate were observed only in response to the spouses' pain displays, and these effects were more powerful where the marriage was satisfactory than where it was not (although the intensity of the pain ratings did not differ between the two situations). In that empathy between partners may be regarded as one of the defining characteristics of marriages that work, such a finding was perhaps predictable. In certain circumstances leaving the marriage might be construed as a healthy response, depending on the level of commitment. Alternatively, the chronic pain patient may come to appreciate that the partner's tolerance can be stretched only so far, and thus he or she may learn to restrain excessive demands in time to save the marriage. *A priori* we can assume that there is often plenty of room for manoeuvre, whatever the shortage of empirical data.

Confirmation of the crucial role of the spouse is to be found in a report by Swanson and Maruta (1980). Routine use of a simple twenty-one-item questionnaire with pain patients admitted to the Mayo Clinic led them to the fortuitous observation of a strange paradox. The greater the congruence between the patient's responses and those of the next of kin (usually a spouse but sometimes a parent or other relative), the poorer the outcome on follow-up after discharge from the clinic. The questionnaire encompassed the nature and severity of the pain, its effect on sleep, mood, work, recreation, and sexual life, factors which aggravated or relieved it, and so forth. Most of the patients were back pain sufferers, and though the degree of chronicity was variable there had been limited response to conventional therapy. The authors interpreted their curious finding in terms of an 'undesirable mutuality', such that the patient's progress was evidently hampered by undue vigilance on the home front. Whilst this modest study needs to be replicated before it can be taken too seriously, it does appear to extend the concept of marital collusion to other close relationships. Parents, of course, have an incorrigible urge to fuss over their sick children even when they come of age, and the parent–child relationship is not uncommonly a model for the first marital relationship. It can take a lifetime to work a parent out of one's system, and it is perfectly normal to re-enact the parental role from time to time in marriage. However, what may be harmless enough in a state of health can become ultimately destructive in a state of sickness.

The need for marital assessment

A case can be made for involving the partner soon after the referral of a chronic pain patient who is married or stably cohabiting. Clinicians may have been slow to realize this, and much of the earlier literature on pain management betrays little or no awareness of the role of the spouse; however, there have been several attempts in recent years to redress the balance by applying psychodynamic or behavioural concepts to the study of chronic pain in a marital context (e.g. Delvey and Hopkins 1982; Waring 1982; Block and Boyer 1984; Ahern *et al*. 1985; Rowat and Knafl 1985; Flor, Kerns, and Turk 1987; Flor, Turk, and Scholz 1987). But even before the emergence of these review articles, which demonstrate the relevance of looking beyond the individual patient without detailed evidence as to the possible therapeutic gains, Fordyce and his colleagues in Seattle had already shown what can be achieved through behavioural and marital re-education where medicine and surgery had little to offer. Their detailed case report (Fordyce *et al*. 1968) laid no undue stress on the contribution of the spouse, yet it was plainly indispensable.

Mrs Y was a 37-year-old high school graduate with a 'bright, upward mobile husband' who worked as a school administrator, and a teenage son. Since 1948, about a year after her marriage, she had suffered from virtually constant low back pain and had become gradually less capable of running her home. On admission to the medical rehabilitation department of a teaching hospital she was complaining of continuous backache which increased with activity of any kind. She needed a rest period every 20 minutes even when actively engaged in a task, and according to her husband she would spend all but about two hours of her normal day reading, watching television or sleeping. Whenever her pain was exacerbated she would take medication and cry until it subsided, thereby eliciting much sympathy from both husband and son.

Between 1951 and 1962 she had undergone four surgical procedures, the most recent of which was a spinal fusion. Technically these were judged to have been successful, and there was no evidence of any neurological deficit, yet her pain persisted. In hospital a treatment schedule was devised to maintain healthier behaviour and enhance her general level of activity. Medication was given at fixed intervals rather than when she complained of pain, and within six weeks of admission the narcotic content was reduced to zero (unknown to either patient or nursing staff). All staff members were instructed to be as unresponsive as possible to her complaints of pain and discomfort whilst reacting positively to all signs of activity, especially when increased over the previous day. Thus 'pain behaviour received a minimum of reinforcement while activity was maximally reinforced' (p. 105). In addition, an occupational therapy programme was introduced with rest as the reinforcer. She was also given a notebook for recording all unscheduled activities to the nearest minute, and she was seen daily to construct progress graphs from her own records. Her response to eight weeks of rehabilitation was quite dramatic.

We can doubtless accept the authors' claim that judicious use of three potential reinforcers available in medical settings – medication, rest, and social attention – will produce significant effects on pain behaviour (Fordyce *et al.* 1968: 107). The drawback of such programmes is that relapse can be anticipated after return to the normal environment where the modifying influences are no longer operating. This problem was tackled through weekly meetings between the psychologist and the husband, who was asked to monitor his wife's weekend activities according to the same principles of behaviour modification. She was thereby enabled to extend her performance in various ways, socially and domestically. Even so, she relapsed when she got home and had to be seen regularly as an out-patient for six months. During this immediate follow-up period she regained her new-found level of activity, and thereafter she was seen only at monthly intervals for a brief check on progress. Meanwhile the purchase of a second car had allowed her to start driving lessons with a view to promoting her independence and mobility in the local community.[1]

This case history demonstrates that all is not necessarily lost even after repeated surgical failure. It has already been pointed out that only a minute proportion of back sufferers get as far as the operating table, yet it is precisely those whose pain is resistant to other therapeutic measures over many years who are most likely to be considered for surgery. By this time the patient will have become firmly entrenched in the invalid role, so that behavioural measures may be needed as an important part of after-care even where the indications for operating are clear-cut. Ideally a behavioural re-education programme of the kind described calls for residential facilities, and it is a matter of lasting regret that there are so few centres in Britain at the present time where such a programme could be launched with any realistic hope of success.

A factor that must be carefully weighed in planning any treatment programme that makes demands upon the patient's family is the personality of the spouse. Attitudes to the marriage must be explored, and it may be equally vital to appraise how he or she views the helping professions in general as well as the specific regime proposed. Half-hearted co-operation will be of no avail, and emotional stability of a high order may be required. We are told all too little about the husband in the case just quoted, but he must have exercised quite astonishing forbearance throughout almost twenty years of ruined marriage. Such remarkably loyal partners are likely to be rare; commoner by far are men with feet of clay, as in a case fully reported elsewhere (Humphrey 1985) and briefly recapitulated here.

A woman of 35 was admitted to the Wolfson Medical Rehabilitation Centre for the second time. Eight years earlier she had fallen on her own doorstep, and despite normal X-ray findings she soon became a chronic pain patient. Shortly after her discharge from the centre she had a combined laminectomy and spinal fusion, after which she went steadily from bad to worse. Her husband took over most of the household management, which may have suited him well enough in view of his self-avowed need to be the dominant partner. He implied in casual conversation at our first meeting that power was more gratifying to him than sex, which owing to the intensity of her pain had come to play only a minor part in their marriage.

The couple were visited at home several times for both joint and separate discussions of their problem, and she was persuaded to keep a pain diary for five consecutive weeks. This showed a good deal of avoidance behaviour which ought to have been open to modification, yet his manipulative behaviour in which she appeared to collude was an effective barrier to re-education. The mutually destructive aspects of their relationship were cause for concern, especially after he had forgone promotion in the police force and lost substantial income in order that he could spend more time with her. She had been treated by a psychiatrist in the past and still suffered from depression. The outlook for this functionally crippled semi-invalid woman was scarcely reassuring, with her daughter fast growing up and not much prospect of resuming even part-time work to escape from her domestic frustrations.

When seen later at the clinic she explained that her normally

attentive husband was 'unable to get away', but as it
happened we already knew that he was serving a prison
sentence for corruption in the course of duty. At her most
recent visit she was more honest, perhaps because she had at
last been given the opportunity to rely on her own resources.

This bald summary may suggest that the initial therapeutic plan
was excessively optimistic, yet the sequence of events was slow to
unfold. In assessing a marriage with a view to enlisting the partner's co-operation there is indeed no substitute for clinical skill;
and regrettably the use of marital questionnaires (e.g. Ryle 1966;
Spanier 1976) is heavily dependent on the degree of co-operation
on offer. In this case there was mounting evidence of the husband's hostility lurking behind a façade of goodwill.

Pain and sexuality

A recurrent problem in the lives of chronic pain patients is loss
of sexual interest and impairment of performance. Obviously this
is not confined to married or cohabiting patients, and the immediate handicap may be all the greater in the absence of a steady
partnership. Thus a 35-year-old divorced man participating in a
discussion group at the Wolfson Centre caused some amusement
by recalling how a newly acquired girlfriend had refused to believe
him when he was compelled by his pain to leave her stranded in
mid-act. However, it cannot have been funny for either of them
at the time. Marriage itself after the onset of intractable pain is
unlikely to be rare, yet the tribulations of courtship are inevitably
increased. The intrusion of sexual difficulties into long-term
relationships can have even more damaging consequences. Much
will depend on the stage at which this happens, and we have
already noted that most of our clinic patients are middle-aged and
thus likely on average to have been married for twenty years or
more. This does not dispose of all the anguish but it does effectively reduce the risk of complete marital disruption.

Maruta and Osborne (1978), in the first of two reports from the
Mayo Clinic, noted that almost two-thirds of a group of sixty-six
married patients acknowledged a decline in their sexual adjustment, whilst more than a third regarded the marriage itself as
adversely affected. As the authors observe:

This does not mean that these patients have clinically significant problems. Rather it means that, after the onset of the pain problem, more than half the patients with chronic pain experienced definite changes in their sexual adjustment which were significant enough to be discussed when an opportunity was provided.

(Maruta and Osborne 1978: 533)

In a further study of 25 male and 25 female patients (mean age 43, range 20–64), most of whom were complaining of pain in the back or extremities if not both, good agreement was found between patient and spouse on the reduction of coital frequency and satisfaction (Maruta *et al*. 1981). Pain after sexual activity was a common occurrence, as was its recognition by the partner. Difficulty in reaching orgasm was a problem for only four women before the onset of pain but for ten women thereafter. None of the men recalled sexual inadequacies of any kind prior to their pain, whereas almost a third reported premature ejaculation or difficulty in achieving or sustaining an erection once the pain had become established. Previous marital adjustment was rated as satisfactory by 80 per cent of both patients and spouses, whereas three times as many spouses as patients (54 per cent versus 18 per cent) rated their adjustment over the last six months as below average. This suggests a degree of defensiveness on the part of the patients, who may have felt uneasy about their role in the loss of marital intimacy. On the other hand some of the difficulty may well have arisen from the partner's fear of inflicting pain, as with the husband of the woman described in Chapter 2 (p. 25). It should not be forgotten that sexual intercourse is supposed to be pleasurable, and to persist with it in a state of pain may come to seem like a travesty for both partners.

Patients referred from the back pain clinic for psychological assessment are seldom ready to maintain that all is well with the sexual side of marriage. In a few instances sex had always been a problem, but even allowing for an element of retrospective distortion it seems reasonable to assume that the majority of couples presenting at such a clinic will have functioned well enough for ordinary purposes prior to the onset of chronic pain. Interestingly, they appear disinclined to ask for help, with a few notable exceptions. Young men and women undergoing rehabilitation at the Wolfson Centre are perhaps more likely to ask to see the psychologist for this purpose, but middle age is evidently a time for beginning to come to terms with a decline in sexual interest and activity. Often the unimpaired partner, whether male or female, will insist in response to a direct question that he or she is 'not worried' about this aspect of marriage.

Pain and the family

Although variables relating to family interaction are notoriously hard to pinpoint in a research design, there has at least been a recent growth of interest in reviewing what is already known (e.g. Roy 1982; Payne and Norfleet 1986; Turk *et al.* 1987; Flor, Turk, and Rudy 1987). It is generally agreed that chronic pain in one member of a nuclear family is almost certain to make an impact on other members. What is much less clear is whether – and if so how far – family events and relationships can give rise to chronic pain. It is equally open to debate whether family members should routinely be involved in the management of individual pain problems. Doubts may be raised as to the cost-effectiveness of such a policy, which might be hard to implement anyway. What might be called the family therapy movement – pioneered by American workers such as Satir (1967) and Minuchin (1974) – has obviously come to stay, but controlled studies of outcome have been rare indeed. And in the sphere of chronic pain they are nonexistent.

In a recent review of the literature, Turk, Flor and Rudy (1987) look at evidence bearing on the question of whether family processes can trigger or help to perpetuate chronic pain in a family member. They are also concerned with the impact of chronic pain in one member upon others, which is not such a difficult issue to investigate. Even so, controlled research studies of this last aspect are remarkably scant, and most of the relevant material is descriptive in nature. A report by Richards *et al.* (1980) has shown the way by assessing various social and psychological as well as medical factors in seventy-five victims of pain arising from spinal cord injuries. Pain intensity and intrusiveness were found to be affected by variables relating to the family, and patients fared worse when living in a more difficult environment (as rated by three social workers independently). This finding should cause no surprise even if it was well worth demonstrating. More helpful perhaps would be a comparison of those whose pain was due to a clearly defined lesion (as in this case) and those where it was of more obscure origin (as in the majority of chronic patients). For although personal and interpersonal factors may contribute to the cause of paraplegia in particular instances, as already argued, they are far more likely to relate to lumbar pain of non-traumatic origin. An enquiry along these lines would be less beset by obstacles than the more ambitious efforts of research-minded family therapists.

The fact that chronic disease and disability must by definition extend over time is reason enough for exploring the contribution of family members, whether positive or negative (Litman 1974; Litman and Venters 1979). When we consider the typical patient with chronic pain, implications for the family are not hard to discern. As Turk *et al.* (1987: 4) point out:

> Many have lost gainful employment, rely on disability payments or have to live on their spouse's earnings, and thus experience considerable financial strains. Pain and disability may lead to mood alterations in the patient that can adversely affect the family that has to deal with altered roles and responsibilities.

Behavioural scientists have been known to fall into the trap of ignoring or underplaying socioeconomic factors which can make such an enormous difference to the individual family's resources for coping with illness or disablement, be it sudden and severe or insidious and of uncertain outlook. Financial solvency is plainly no guarantee against disturbed relationships between partners or between parents and children, but it must surely help to cushion the shock and mitigate the worst of the long-term effects. Hence a broad perspective becomes essential and is probably best achieved through interdisciplinary collaboration. Moreover it is inappropriate to focus exclusively on the spouse, however far-reaching his or her role. In our own work to date we have tended to do so, purely as a matter of convenience. Other members of the family do turn up at the clinic from time to time even when the patient is married, occasionally to act as interpreter where there are language difficulties but more often for no obvious reason. A new angle is thus afforded, and a case could be made for seeking to involve other relatives more often, especially as so few of our patients live alone. In the management of a clinical service this is partly a question of time, whereas research workers are under no such constraints.

Both from patients who attend our back pain clinic over an extended period and from those who are rehabilitated at the Wolfson Centre (usually for up to a month at a stretch), we have learnt a great deal informally about the complex interplay of marital and other factors that can influence the outcome. Adequate and discreet support – as supposed to hostility, over-protection, or reinforcement of pain behaviour – is an asset that needs careful evaluation even if it remains hard to measure. A notable consequence of this wider perspective is that surgery for the relief of intractable pain has become almost a rare event, despite the fact that our clinic was established and is organized by an orthopaedic surgeon. At the present time no more than 5–10 per cent of our clientele are offered surgery, and almost invariably the offer is accepted. What we still lack are the necess-ary resources for implementing alternative styles of management on behalf of the other 90–95 per cent. Few clinical psychologists are interested and available to absorb any of the load, and an inescapable feature of work with families is that it is time-consum-ing. Future prospects will be discussed in the final chapter.

In lamenting the lack of valid and reliable instruments for assessing how families function, Flor *et al.* (1987) nevertheless argue that family members should be involved in any treatment plan. Yet they also draw attention to the absence of agreed criteria for embarking on family therapy as such, and plead for more and better research. However, in view of the notorious difficulties of researching into family processes there is probably something to be said for relying on clinical judgement rather than waiting for the cautious recommendations of research workers, which may be of little practical help. Often enough it is crystal clear that interpersonal factors of one sort or another are impeding the resolution of chronic pain, as in the following case. A Wolfson patient aged 26 was looking for a sex therapist (*sic*). His story was that he had almost given up working as a self-employed decorator over the past year because it was taking him so long to finish anything. This meant that his girlfriend was having to take over responsibility for the substantial mortgage payments on his maisonette, where she visited him daily – she did not live with him. Their sexual relationship had indeed declined for some while prior to his laminectomy nearly three months before, and after the operation she had been obliged to act as nursemaid in the bathroom. He had been sent home within ten days of the operation when he was still uncertain of his ability to care for himself. In this stressful situation he not surprisingly lost confidence in his power to retain the young woman's affections, and began trying to make love to her before he was ready for this. Within a short time of his discharge from the rehabilitation centre the relationship ended stormily, and when last seen his pain was clearly exacerbated by his sense of failure in both love and work.

The hazards of over-enthusiastic treatment

It is reassuring to find that clinicians and researchers alike have become aware that intervening in a marriage according to the dictates of an operant model is not without risk. Encouraging the spouse to ignore complaints of pain while rewarding signs of activity can easily disturb the balance of an uneasy equilibrium. In their study of psychogenic pain, Hughes et al. (1987) found that the spouses of fifteen pain patients had a better marital adjustment and less psychiatric morbidity than the spouses of a matched group of neurotic patients attending the same department. This finding was paradoxical in that the pain patients displayed rather more impairment in their social, sexual, and occupational roles than the neurotic patients, and were manifestly over-dependent on their partners in daily life. The authors had recourse to an explanation in terms of 'sick role homeostasis' (Waring 1977) and 'tertiary gain' (Bokan et al. 1981). It was as if the pain was somehow holding the marriage together by providing a common focus and an escape from conflict in the relationship.

Sternbach (1974) and more especially Szasz (1968) have dwelt on the art of 'painmanship', which refers to the use of pain as a weapon of interpersonal control. This brings us back to the question of enhanced marital stability which appears to typify the chronic pain patient. Careful enquiry has revealed that for many married couples attending the St George's back pain clinic, the effects of pain and its associated disability are all-pervasive. When first seen at least 50 per cent of both men and women either were unemployed, were on sick leave, or had taken early retirement; domestic chores had been reassigned and leisure pursuits were severely curtailed (Humphrey and Jones 1987). One would surely expect pain of these dimensions to play havoc with a relationship if not to destroy it. Yet this had not happened, even if the pain had come to dominate the relationship. It is hard to avoid the assumption that these couples were in some way continuing to meet one another's emotional needs, albeit in a self-defeating manner.

Reluctance to abandon a stricken partner could be one factor in the survival of these marriages, especially when the marriage was strongly established long before the onset of pain. Loyalty on the part of the healthy spouse has been observed often enough in other contexts, such as stroke (Coughlan and Humphrey 1982). Even so, there are significant differences between gross physical disablement following a sudden catastrophe, and pain which is commonly of insidious onset and open to a psychosomatic interpretation. Where abnormal illness behaviour is a prominent feature, as in so many of the more intractable cases of back pain, the risk of marital breakdown ought really to be greater than for pain-free couples at the same stage of the life-cycle. Whilst we cannot afford to underestimate a healthy individual's capacity for adapting to invalidism in a spouse, we must also remain alert to the struggle for power which some of these couples may be enacting before our very eyes. And if a perfectly fit husband or wife is willing to capitulate to the demands of a sick partner then we need to understand why.

There is often no way out of this kind of impasse. Confronting the parties to a collusive marriage can be hazardous, as already indicated, and should be left to experienced therapists. Sometimes all that can be offered is a listening ear during periods of increased stress, should the couple wish to avail themselves of it. But the chances are that they will be wholly committed to the pursuit of a conventional cure, in the everlasting hope that a series of direct onslaughts on the pain will ultimately do the trick. In this they are doomed to disappointment. Thus Bokan *et al.* (1981), on the basis of three case reports, were led to a rather sober conclusion:

> The difficulty . . . is that patients are presenting themselves
> for treatment of their pain, they would like to be rid of it;
> however, they are unwilling to give up the advantages accrued
> from the pain (primary and/or secondary gain). This scene
> is further complicated by the effect of persons other than the
> patient who may be unwilling to give up the advantages they

have obtained from the patient's pain problems (tertiary gain). To make matters even more difficult, in the authors' experience, most of these gains involve an unconscious or non-volitional mechanism.

(Bokan *et al.* 1981: 334)

When attention is also given to the incidental advantages accruing to the physicians, surgeons, and others who set out to treat chronic pain (especially under the American health care system), it becomes obvious why therapeutic success has proved so elusive.

Chapter four

Work, leisure activities, and social life

Even if the majority of chronic pain patients are married or cohabiting, there will always be some who are living alone for whatever reason. Deprived of the far-reaching commitment of marriage and family life, or having in some cases chosen to forgo it, such individuals may have come to depend more heavily on work as a major source of satisfaction. By the same token they may have invested more wholeheartedly in leisure pursuits, be they social or solitary. Hence the impact of their pain problem may be even more devastating, especially if (as in a few cases) they have nobody with whom to share it or who can help to cushion them against its worst effects. When we recognize also that married people have been known to use an absorbing career or hobbies as a bulwark against the demands of family life at its most intrusive, or as a retreat from the declining intimacies of a failed relationship, then it seems appropriate to pay particular attention to the effects of long-term handicap on work and leisure activities.

In order to lend substance to our discussion a series of 50 clinic attenders, drawn in alphabetical sequence from my case load over the past three years, have been analysed from this standpoint. They comprise 29 women and 21 men, of whom 38 were currently married and another three cohabiting. Their mean age was 44.5, with a range of 21–68; only 2 men and 3 women were under 30, in keeping with the usual pattern at this clinic. A man and 4 women had a history of spinal surgery; one of the women had experienced many years of relief from pain, whereas 2 others had undergone a second operation without lasting benefit. Thirteen men and 22 working women were unemployed at the time of their first attendance, and few are known to have found employment (ideally in the form of a lighter job) during an average follow-up period of around 18 months. Age distribution, marital status, fitness for work, and level of employment were comparable for men and women. Only 1 man and 2 women were graduates with professional qualifications, although 2 other women were State Registered Nurses. Illustrative material from this small sample will be used throughout this chapter as and where appropriate.

Pacers versus recliners: an operant view of pain behaviour

Before looking in detail at the kind of lives these patients were leading, inside and outside the home, it may be helpful to introduce a means towards conceptual clarification that can be credited to Fordyce (1976). Having noted that chronic pain victims, already trapped by their physical problems, could become still further handicapped by their attitudes to these problems, Fordyce went on to distinguish between two extreme types. *Pacers* were those who had learnt that they could gain relief from their pain through movement. They therefore refused to capitulate to it, neither moderating their activities nor accepting sensible limitations. These are the patients who – in my experience – insist on digging the garden, for example, knowing full well that they would bitterly regret their foolhardiness the following day and probably for several days thereafter; or they would continue painting a vast expanse of ceiling long after their bodily signals had been urging them to desist. There are some tasks that may be safely attempted by the chronic back pain sufferer, and others that should be delegated to their more fortunate brethren. This is not a matter of evasion but of prudent avoidance – if they persist they will not only have cause to rue it, they may also succeed in making life difficult for their nearest and dearest by being laid up when their services are most needed. In other words, they are prone to what another psychologist has referred to as 'injudicious bursts of activity' (Jones 1985: 10). There is no merit in contriving one's own frustration even if most of us do it from time to time, and here there is ample scope for preventive counselling.

A totally different hazard is incurred by *recliners*, who are so fearful of doing themselves harm that they are apt to fight shy of even the most innocent pastimes. This kind of pain victim is prone to 'avoidance behaviour', in the sense used by clinical psychologists, i.e. they deprive themselves of ordinary learning opportunities that might enable them to overcome their difficulties at least in part. They turn up at the back pain clinic rather more often than pacers, or it may be that they are more easily recognized. (The policeman described in Chapter 2, p. 28, is a case in point. On a subsequent visit he confessed to a perfectly understandable fear of physical assault.) Such patients can be helped, although not primarily by conventional medicine or surgery. The use of behavioural re-education programmes has been illustrated in the previous chapter, and there can be little doubt that the disabled housewife whose case was summarized on pp. 38–9 (see Fordyce *et al.* 1968) was a recliner rather than a pacer.

This crude dichotomy cannot hope to embrace all the nuances of human behaviour under stress, and a further difficulty is that chronic pain sufferers tend to fluctuate between the two extremes. As Jones (1985) observed from his exploratory study of twenty-five patients undergoing rehabilitation at the Wolfson Centre, the same person can be a recliner in some circumstances and a pacer in others. Human beings are not entirely consistent in their day-to-day performance, and this has always been one of the major problems faced by behavioural scientists. But in clinical practice it may be helpful, in a preliminary discussion of how to live with pain, to refer to these contrasted forms of maladaptive behaviour. It is not easy to determine which of these biases poses the greater hazard to normal living. On balance it might be considered more hopeful to err in the direction of over-activity, not only because this is likely to be a sign of a more robust personality but also because under-activity may be less readily open to modification. However, this remains somewhat speculative and therefore unreliable as a guide to rehabilitation. For this purpose we need systematic studies of individual patterns of activity over a time span, ideally with the help of pain diaries as well as controlled observation.

The distinction between pacers and recliners was one that emerged naturally from Fordyce's behaviourist philosophy. This had led him not only to play down the traditional medical model with its emphasis on physiological aberration and disease processes, but also to reject alternative models that laid stress on unconscious mechanisms or deep-seated personality traits. To counteract these inadequate or outmoded approaches he urged

that more cognizance be taken of *learning theory* in the explanation of pain that defied medical or surgical treatment. To this
end he distinguished between *respondent* pain and *operant* pain.
Respondent pain refers to that which is rooted in a specific noxious
stimulus (e.g. arising from known tissue damage), whereas operant pain is viewed as an outcome of reinforcement derived from
environmental contingencies. Whilst conceding that most chronic
pain problems were likely to have originated as respondent pain
following an organic lesion, Fordyce contended that often enough
when the tissue damage had been repaired the pain nevertheless
persisted with much the same quality (if not the same intensity)
because it was being maintained by factors in the sufferer's
environment. Thus chronic pain was particularly vulnerable to the
effects of incidental learning.

Fordyce has been widely criticized for his somewhat cavalier
attitude towards pain experience, which after all is the whole basis
of the patient's complaint. He has indeed tended to focus on
quantifiable 'pain behaviour', which comprises not only verbal
expressions but 'all audible and visible displays of pain-related
suffering, such as gasps, moans, sighs, grimacing, limping, guard-
ing, bracing and so on' (Jones 1985: 8). It is not hard to understand
the appeal of such a concrete model to many clinical psychologists,
who will have applied it with varying success in the treatment of
other maladaptive behaviours. It is undoubtedly oversimplified,
but has been brought in here as a means of sharpening the reader's
perspective on pain management as it relates to activity level. For
even when the patient's complaints continue unabated, provided
that some semblance of normal activity has been restored we can
begin to speak of partial recovery. The more active the sufferer,
in other words, the better his or her morale; and it is reasonable
to suppose that improved morale will help to diminish the intensity
of pain. Obviously there are some chronic disorders (rheumatoid
arthritis, for instance) for which such an approach would be
impracticable or unwise, if not downright dangerous. However, it
can be stated with some confidence that the commonest types of
back pain are not among them. And even respondent pain such
as that due to ankylosing spondylitis, which starts as a progressive
disorder, need not preclude a behavioural approach. Whatever
the aetiology of their pain problem, most patients stand to gain
from gently increased activity even if at first it has to be under
close medical supervision.

Involvement in a graded programme of activity at a rehabilitation centre can have immediately beneficial effects. Thus Fordyce *et al.* (1978) found that chronic pain patients who recorded more time spent walking were less depressed and generally less disturbed on the MMPI than those who walked less. The relationship between level of activity and intensity of pain is apparently less close than many pain patients like to assume. A study of thirty back pain sufferers referred consecutively to a medical centre in Sweden found evidence of marked individual variation in the link between level of reported pain and level of activity as measured by self-monitoring or observed behaviour in a test situation (cycling to tolerance). 'Avoidance of certain activities seems to be related more to anxiety and fear about pain than to an actual pain–activity relationship' (Linton 1985: 293).

The possible advantages of remaining at work, or of returning to work after a spell of sick leave, should be considered in the light of this observation. Folkard *et al.* (1976), working at the Abingdon Pain Relief Clinic, found that both men and women who went out to work recorded a decrease in pain intensity during the morning which remained fairly constant until the early evening; and even after returning home they seemed to experience less pain than the group who stayed at home all day. Pain ratings were derived from visual analogue scales, which other workers (e.g. Scott and Huskisson 1976; Price *et al.* 1983) have found satisfactory. Numbers were small (18 versus 23), and no details are given of the kind of work involved which is likely to be crucial in the individual case. However, this report bears out clinical experience of the demoralizing effects on patients of being stuck at home with nothing much to distract them from their pain. This applies particularly to labourers used to heavy manual work who have had to give up the unequal struggle, yet have no realistic prospects of tackling a clerical job even if they were able to countenance the idea (which most are not).

Work

In what follows, the central importance of work for many of our patients and their frustration at being unable to remain employed will need to be borne in mind. Some have lost very little working time, others have endured longish spells of sick leave, while others again have been unemployed for months or years on end. Often their prospects of resuming work were uncertain, sometimes bleak. Among the male patients seven were registered as unemployed and one had retired at a normal age. A computer analyst who had been contemplating a new career in his mid-forties had worked only fitfully and in a reduced capacity since being involved in a head-on collision as a minicab driver. Of the remaining 12 patients, nine had been off work for less than a year (range 3–9 months) and the other three had not worked for two years, three years and seven years respectively, although apparently not yet registered as unemployed. Occupations were varied, including policeman (3), prison officer, ambulance attendant, electrician, paint-sprayer, long-distance lorry driver, newsagent, and aquatic dealer. Some 40 per cent of the women were housewives with family responsibilities, and several of these were still managing to work part-time outside the home. Others had grown-up children, and a relatively high proportion of married women (about one in five) were childless even if in one or two instances this was not necessarily to be so for life. The meaning of prolonged unemployment can be different for married women, who may find it easier to compromise for the sake of their domestic role. Of the eight who had not worked for a year or more, one or two had settled for early retirement but none was without regrets. The saddest case was an unmarried vet in her late fifties who had not practised for at least seven years.

A wide range of attitudes to the non-working man's role was encountered, as would be expected in any random series of households. At one extreme was complete role reversal, which seemed more likely to occur where there were young children. A prison officer and his wife provided a good example of this mutual adaptability.

The man in question was 35 when first seen. He had been injured in the course of riot squad training, about a year after his remarriage to a younger woman who had also been married before. He had custody of the three children from his first marriage, whose ages ranged from 4 to 9 at the time of the accident. A child of the present marriage was born within a month of the accident, much against the couple's original expectations as the wife was convinced of her infertility. At the latest follow-up appointment she was demonstrating her competence as a shop manageress, and he appeared fully reconciled to running the home and caring for the children, of whom the youngest was now approaching school age.

He had returned to modified duties for a while but was then retired from the prison service on medical grounds, with a disability pension of 15 per cent which was due shortly for review by the DHSS. His MMPI profile was normal and apparently reliable, despite unmistakable signs of pain behaviour both at the initial consultation and subsequently. All the evidence suggested that he was enjoying his role as a househusband-cum-father, displaying a good deal of versatility given that he could pace himself and avoid undue strain on his lumbar spine. The effect on the marriage was hard to gauge but there had been little time for the couple to develop set habits before the accident.

Another factor promoting this short-term solution was the patient's jaundiced view of his first marriage, the failure of which he attributed at least partly to his irregular hours as a prison officer. The departure from convention in the present relationship had advantages for both parties. His honourable discharge from the prison service had conferred protection from the risk of further injury, whilst she could make her escape during working hours from all the usual domestic irritations which can be so easily compounded by step-parenthood.

At the opposite extreme was the following situation.

A Post Office supervisor aged 51 had developed back trouble after falling from a ladder some 10 years earlier. The pain had gradually got worse, but he had sought no advice until six months before attending the back pain clinic. At that stage he had woken up one morning unable to move, and was seen by my orthopaedic colleague in Harley Street. A few months after the initial meeting at the clinic he produced an MMPI profile that was atypical of the chronic pain patient and more reminiscent of the psychiatric out-patient clinic. By now he had been off work for eight months on the grounds that he could not cope with sitting.

A recent medical examination on behalf of the Post Office (for which he had worked since leaving school, with no known complaints on either side) had raised doubts about his prolonged sick leave, and I was approached by the DHSS for a psychiatric opinion. There was no record of formal psychiatric illness, but the request was side-stepped as inappropriate to be handled by a psychologist. It may be of some relevance that he had been at risk of over-protection as an only child with asthma, and had spent periods in hospital for other reasons also; and his loyal wife might well have been acting maternally towards him now that their own only child had established his independence. There was no indication that he was pulling his weight domestically whilst on sick leave, and when next seen the couple were plainly resentful about the pressure that was being put on him to return to work. We later referred him to a psychiatric colleague, who concurred with our own view of his self-induced disability.

Between these extremes of active adaptation and passive acceptance were a wide range of responses to the enforced loss of activity, or perhaps it is begging the question to describe it in such terms. Certainly there were men and women who continued to struggle heroically with taxing jobs when given the option, but rarely was there any need to advise a patient to give up work for strictly medical reasons. Workers who had been engaged in heavy manual work had invariably made this decision for themselves, and it was only in more ambiguous situations that attitudes and behavioural style had come to play a major part in determining how a patient would cope with work-related stresses. Where grounds for recommending sick leave appear flimsy, it has been our policy to draw attention to the psychological consequences of prolonged unemployment, knowing that weeks can so readily stretch into months. Speedy resumption of work after short periods of exacerbation can help to prevent secondary handicap, and many patients of either sex are uneasily aware of the need to keep working if at all possible. However, it would be unwise to pronounce judgement on fitness for work without a careful analysis of what the job entails. The pain-racked receptionist may find it increasingly hard to manage awkward customers, or the ageing clerk may balk at reaching down to the bottom drawer of a filing cabinet. Travelling to work can present problems too, as with the young Wolfson patient who did not trust himself to back the car out of his garage, let alone drive it a few miles to the major conurbation where until eight months previously he had been in charge of a shoe shop. Getting to work can be stressful enough for the physically fit, whether at the wheel on today's crowded roads or by public transport.

Room for manoeuvre in the workplace is what the chronic pain patient needs but does not always get. Gross dissatisfaction with working life may have contributed to the pain problem in some instances, with boredom as perhaps the main enemy. Findings which point in this direction were reported by Magora (1973) from a study of selected occupations in Israel: clerks, bus drivers, policemen, nurses, farmers, and workers in light or heavy industry. Dissatisfaction with present work emerged more often in back pain sufferers, regardless of the degree of physical stress involved. Some jobs are inherently soul-destroying, yet even professional qualifications cannot ensure a sense of vocation. The occasional doctor will turn up as a patient, and one such who had been diagnosed as depressed by a senior partner was unable to practice for months on end, ostensibly on account of his pain. He appeared somewhat ill at ease in the medical profession and might well have gained greater satisfaction in some other walk of life.

It is not usually our place to offer vocational guidance, especially to the individual in a well-established career, but persistent pain can sometimes be construed as a symbol of precarious adjustment to the demands of working life. It has often been remarked that a happy marriage is one of the most effective antidotes to stressful experience, but a congenial job can perform much the same function. And it is unfortunate that even comparatively minor disability can pinpoint the weaknesses in an individual's overall adjustment to life.

Leisure activities

As part of the psychological assessment procedure, patients are asked to complete two pencil-and-paper questionnaires as well as the MMPI. These are the Oswestry Scale (Fairbank *et al.* 1980), which was designed specifically to measure the interference of low back pain with daily activities, and the Pain Avoidance Scale (Humphrey and McNally 1983).

The Oswestry Scale has not been adequately standardized even with spinal patients, but no better instrument could be found for our purposes at the time. It comprises ten sections, each with a choice of six responses indicating progressive impairment. After extended use its value has become enhanced, and despite one or two minor blemishes which are open to amendment we shall probably continue to rely on it for a detailed picture of what does and does not cause difficulty to the patient. The Pain Avoidance Scale is a more ambitious tool for attempting to measure the discrepancy between frequency (not quality) of performance when pain-free and when pain is at its worst. It comprises ten social and ten domestic items to be rated on a four-point scale ranging from 0 = 'seldom or never' to 3 = 'very often'. A considerable body of data has accumulated since the first experimental version was devised in 1983, but it has remained unpublished until now partly owing to problems of interpretation. For example, some patients find it hard to recall what life was like when free of pain, having suffered intermittently if not more or less constantly over the past several years. However, granted that it may be hazardous to compare one respondent with another, Jones (1985) reported a satisfactory level of internal consistency for both measures when repeated after an interval of 4–6 weeks' intensive rehabilitation. Reliability coefficients were 0.9 for the Oswestry Scale and more than 0.8 for the Pain Avoidance Scale, apart from the domestic items of the 'pain-free' section.[1] Copies of the two questionnaires are to be found in Appendices I and II.

An item analysis of the Oswestry Scale findings on our fifty patients revealed only minor differences between men and women (Table 4.1). Each item is scored from 0 to 5 according to the degree of interference with daily life, and the maximum score is therefore 50 which makes it easy to calculate an overall percentage. Usually it is more informative to look at the variation between individual items, which can be seen from close inspection of the table. Not surprisingly it is lifting that causes most difficulty for either sex; least trouble arises from personal care and sleeping, which was possibly less predictable. Mean total scores of 43.3 per cent for men and 45.4 per cent for women are not significantly different, but they reflect a substantial loss of freedom to take life as it comes. It will be noted that the scale includes both basic manoeuvres (sitting, standing, walking), which enter into almost all leisure activities, and items of a more global nature (personal care, social life, travelling). Some of the impairments reported in conversation with individual patients are relatively specific, e.g.

inability to put on stockings/socks without help, reluctance to get in and out of a car, and so forth.

Table 4.1 Mean scores for individual Oswestry items on a scale of 0–5

Item	Men (21)	Women (29)
Pain intensity	2.2	2.5
Personal care	1.6	1.2
Lifting	3.0	3.6
Walking	1.9	1.6
Sitting	2.4	2.3
Standing	2.4	3.1
Sleeping	1.4	1.3
Sex life	2.3	2.3
Social life	2.6	2.7
Travelling	2.1	2.3

Useful as the Oswestry Scale has proved as a crude index of disablement, the Pain Avoidance Scale can provide a greater wealth of information. Thus quite apart from individual items, which may confirm or run counter to information derived from other sources, it is often useful to make separate comparisons of social and domestic activities under the two conditions ('no pain' and 'pain at its worst'). There are men and women who seem able to persevere with social activities even when domestically crippled, and vice versa. Even more revealing at times is the reported level of activity when free of pain, which can be abysmally low (witness the middle-aged man whose case history is given on pp. 55–6 who appeared to do nothing other than go to work and visit his widowed father or married son). Some lives are unusually restricted in scope; and whilst it is not always safe to rely on verbal report, in ordinary circumstances it is hard to imagine why anyone would choose to portray themselves as comprehensively idle if they were not.

The Pain Avoidance Scale affords a convenient means of identifying areas of life experience which are relatively vulnerable to pain, though none is altogether immune (Table 4.2). Top of the list come jobs inside and outside the home, which are reported as hampered in nine cases out of ten. Despite repeated protestations from our male patients that they are confirmed do-it-yourself enthusiasts, when overcome by pain it seems that many of them are all too ready to let things slide. This is scarcely a matter for regret in view of the aggravation caused by unwise or untimely demands upon an already strained musculature. House-work is almost equally affected. Outside employment has already been discussed, as has sexual intercourse in the previous chapter. Outings of various kinds are quite severely curtailed, and it becomes common practice to invite visitors to the home (doubtless with less preparation than normally) instead of visiting them. Several of our informants have confessed that they can cheerfully lie down in the presence of visitors at home whereas they might hesitate to do so elsewhere. Shopping poses problems by reason of the lifting involved, especially for women, and a favoured solution is to 'hunt in pairs'. Driving on overcrowded suburban roads is no longer much of a pleasure even for those without back pain, but reluctance to eat out in view of the discomfort of per-ching for long periods on ill-adapted restaurant seats or café chairs could be a deprivation for some families. Finally, a third of the men and half the women were aware of cooking less often when the pain was at its worst, although one man in seven was averse to cooking at the best of times. On the whole, sex differences are of no great magnitude, bearing in mind the smallness of the sample

Table 4.2 Pain Avoidance Scale: incidence of reduced activities when pain is at its worst

Activity	Men (21) %	Women (29) %	Combined (50) %
Indoor jobs	86	96	91
Outdoor jobs	85	95	90
Outside employment	81	88	85
Heavy housework	79	89	85
Sexual intercourse	81	78	80
Light gardening	63	86	76
Going to cinema or theatre	67	78	74
Going to parties or dances	67	72	70
Visiting friends or relatives	62	75	69
Shopping	55	75	67
Car trips for pleasure	48	73	60
Eating out	68	56	59
Inviting visitors	40	64	54
Light housework	20	61	44
Cooking	33	50	43

as well as the traditional contrast between male and female roles. A few items (such as engaging in sports and attending social clubs) have been omitted from the table because there were too many 'not applicable' entries.

Whilst the above analysis has focused on reduction rather than cessation of activities, it is also worth looking at what is most likely to go by the board in conditions of severe pain. Apart from sport, which many people are ready to give up in any case well before middle age, the salient items are eating out and going to the cinema or theatre (abandoned by about two in five and three in five members of our sample respectively). Chronic pain can have the effect of curtailing life to its barest essentials, with ordinary obligations evaded or cut to a minimum and even the simplest of diversions eliminated. What may once have been a varied and even colourful life becomes scaled down to a drab existence, with depression adding to the toll of human misery.

Social life

The distinction between leisure activities and social life is to some extent artificial, with many hobbies serving a social as well as a recreational intent. Altered visiting patterns have already been mentioned, and it would appear that a large number of married couples are forced to cultivate a degree of self-sufficiency after one partner has developed back trouble. Some have always been inclined to close their doors against the outside world, restricting their social interchange to close relatives. The majority of our patients have grown up in the same locality, and remain in close touch with elderly parents and most of their siblings. Links can be maintained without undue effort even when mobility (or sometimes the will to remain mobile) is much impaired. To remain socially active beyond the family, whether through club membership or individual outings, calls for more determination, and it may be tempting to withdraw. Active sports such as tennis, squash, and badminton may be virtually ruled out, and those who have kept up their skills and enthusiasm over the pain-free years are unlikely to relish the spectator role. Even a gentle game of billiards may pose too much of a challenge, not only by reason of the movements involved but because the competitive spirit has been dampened by pain. Avoidance of increased discomfort has come to take priority over the assertion of superior skill. Swimming may be permitted and indeed recommended, yet this is often a solitary pursuit.

Data from the Pain Avoidance Scale can help to illuminate the differential impact on domestic and social activities. Here individual circumstances can be even more influential than personality and attitudes. In contrast to the Post Office executive whose wife was dedicated to the task of making life easy for him, a retired postman of 63 had found himself having to care for a dementing older wife who spent most of her time in bed; he did so with infinite forbearance and good grace, despite the added handicaps of a cardiac complaint and an enlarged prostate which required surgery. When I visited him at home he was coping manfully, though plainly at his wits' end. A letter I sent to the orthopaedic consultant immediately after this visit contains the following excerpt:

> [The wife] is a frail 70-year-old who fractured her femur two years ago and apparently has gone steadily downhill since then. Before Christmas she spent six weeks in a darkened room unable to face life, so that her husband had to do everything for her (as indeed he continues to do). I asked her to walk across the room and she did so in a wobbly fashion. . . . Evidently it took six weeks to summon a psychiatrist from [the local hospital] who has referred her on to a psychogeriatrician at [another hospital] where her appointment is in five weeks' time. . . . She can converse normally and is not grossly amnesic, although I was told that I had caught her on one of her good days. Nevertheless she is clearly a heavy drain on our patient's resources, she has lost weight and gives the impression that she is not long for this world.

A year later the situation was essentially unchanged; if anything the wife was 'not quite as well as she had been' and had recently opted out of her weekly trips to the day centre. The patient's back pain continued but was something he had learnt to live with because he saw no alternative. The two offspring had three youngsters apiece, and only the daughter lived near enough to be of any practical help. Yet somehow this goodhearted stoic had been able to maintain a comfortable home in a pleasant neighbourhood, and the absence of all social life did not seem to worry him unduly. He had mastered a full range of domestic duties, which was probably what kept him going.

Two further illustrations will be given more briefly of patients who, for quite different reasons, had preserved some semblance of domestic efficiency at the expense of their social lives. A printer of 55 had recently separated from his wife, and when first seen was not looking forward to his first winter alone. Yet he was more than equal to the challenge of creating his own home now that he had only himself to satisfy. When seen later at the Wolfson Centre he was setting a formidable example to other patients with his exaggerated air of physical fitness. All that he had originally asked of the surgeon was to be restored to his former prowess as a marathon runner, but he was told that he would need more than a spinal fusion to achieve such an unrealistic aim.

A woman of 56 had been through two divorces in singularly traumatic circumstances, but was sustained by the four children of her first marriage (with whom she enjoyed lastingly close relationships) and nine grandchildren. She had not worked for three years, following an accident at her son's home in which she had fractured a vertebra, and missed the company of her mates at the factory. She had given up dancing, her sole recreation, and felt that living alone had become the only acceptable *modus vivendi*. Fortunately she could cope with all the usual domestic tasks, including household repairs when absolutely necessary.

When performance under maximum duress is expressed as a ratio of performance under optimal conditions, there is virtually no discrepancy between social and domestic scores for either men or women. Mean figures as thus calculated range from 0.44 to 0.48. This is merely a cryptic way of saying that, on average and over a wide area of living, these patients were less than half as active when their pain was at its worst, as compared with their ideal state. Such apparent consistency does of course hide a wealth of individual variation, and some patients were under pressure to remain active on all fronts. A former catering manager of 47, though temporarily unemployed, was kept endlessly busy at the behest of his male partner. He was fearful of losing the older man's respect, and could not bring himself to turn away a constant stream of visitors from overseas. His pain had been bothering him intermittently for several years, and was not appreciably relieved during the 18 months or more that he attended the clinic. Yet he had learnt to cope with it after a fashion, with possibly some help from psychological counselling that was also addressed to his drinking problem. His ratios were 0.74 for the domestic and 0.87 for the social items of the scale. He was well motivated to keep going at all costs, and so he did.

Clinical experience suggests that social relationships can be at least partially preserved if the individual has invested wholeheartedly in them before the onset of pain. Withdrawal is most conspicuous among those whose energies have long been primarily committed to routine maintenance and survival, and who may be content with their own company anyway. An invitation from a particularly lively lady to assist in the celebration of her fiftieth birthday was proof that social isolation is not an inevitable consequence of chronic pain, even if many of the other guests were fellow sufferers.[2] Opportunities to observe the back pain victim outside the clinical context have been few and far between, so that due allowance must be made for the clinician's limited perspective. It is easy to develop an exaggerated faith in the accuracy of self-report, and in basing the content of this chapter on what patients say we cannot pretend to be reporting on what they actually do or fail to do.

Giving up the unequal struggle

Even so, a story of greatly reduced activity on all fronts among predominantly middle-aged people, most of whom are currently unable to perform their normal work, rings true in almost every detail. There was usually a partner to verify the patient's own account, and confirmation from other sources such as employers. Despite some convincing examples of magnified pain presentation, for which the evidence was always scrupulously recorded, we doubt whether we were often grossly deceived. The problems presented to us had defied all manner of previous treatments, and the pain syndrome had become chronic by any sensible definition. Many of these hapless individuals had reached a complete impasse in their lives and were seeking rescue from oblivion as well as pain.

What could be done to help them? Therapeutic measures will be discussed more fully in the next two chapters, and here it must suffice to state that our prime concern was to ensure that no obvious steps such as indoctrination in good back care had been overlooked. Some patients insist that nobody had ever tried to teach them how to live with a sensitive back, so that referral to the physiotherapy department becomes an immediate priority. Many patients have been sent for an opinion on the case for spinal surgery, and their expectations are geared to this. Much more often than not they have to be disabused of this notion, and it is ironical that almost as many patients seem to react with disappointment as with relief. Surgery in this context has had a bad press, and when performed on the wrong patient it can leave a devastating aftermath. And although some patients arrive looking towards the surgeon as the wielder of a magic wand that will get rid of their pain once and for all, others have a more sober awareness of the odds against achieving a complete remission in this way. Some 20–30 per cent have already learnt the hard way from previous operations which have conferred no lasting benefit or none at all; and, as already argued, loss of hope in such circumstances is tantamount to deterioration. A spell at a rehabilitation centre is a much safer proposition, for even if it does no good it is unlikely to do any harm. A particular merit of specialized rehabilitation is that it aims at putting the onus of recovery on the patient, fairly and squarely. This, as Broome and Jellicoe (1987) have stressed, is what paves the way to effective self-help.

Helping a chronic pain patient to get back to work is beyond the resources of most clinics, which are not run as employment agencies. To inculcate a more positive approach to life in general, and work in particular, is usually quite hard enough. Enforced inactivity is demoralizing even for those who are idle by nature, and significant improvement can be anticipated from even partial resumption of a more normal lifestyle. If our Post Office supervisor, for example, could have been persuaded to cut short his sick leave, even at the cost of first having to swallow his resentment at being put under pressure, we thought it might have given him a chance to become a healthier as well as a happier human being. This presupposes a correct diagnosis of the problem, and it has to be conceded that sometimes the patient is a better judge than his professional advisors.[3] Rather more commonly, however, there are indications of a massive entrenchment in the invalid role. This can sometimes be tackled, but seldom by direct confrontation.

Which brings us back to Fordyce's operant regime. Chronic pain patients (some but not all) can undoubtedly be helped to become more active; what remains in question is the extent to which their suffering can be relieved, whether in terms of the pain itself or the associated distress. Fordyce himself was less concerned with the subjective element than with the outward and visible signs of rejuvenation – for there are few things more ageing than relentless pain. If there were any obvious means of abolishing the pain then clearly this would constitute the first line of attack, for restoration of normal activities would presumably follow. It is because a variety of methods have been tried and found wanting that the psychologist is invited into the arena. It has been argued previously (Humphrey 1980) that psychologists can earn their keep merely by helping to ward off the surgeon's knife, but as time goes on a lot more is expected of them. Whether they will prove capable of delivering *all* the desired goods awaits further experience, but it seems unlikely. Not for nothing has chronic back pain been regarded as an intractable problem.

Whereas the previous chapter drew heavily on the literature, this one has relied more on clinical experience. Outside the operant framework there has been little enough research on the therapeutic value of activity *per se*, nor on the mood change that may ensue from loss of activity. Two studies by Skevington (1983a, 1983b) provide an exception to this general statement. Working with small groups (n = 14) of rheumatoid arthritis patients, and both patients and ex-patients with pain of unknown origin, she found that the nature and level of their reported activities had some bearing on issues of diagnosis and management. Rheumatoid patients, for example, reported strikingly few recreational activities, as might have been predicted. In her second study she addressed the question of personal versus universal helplessness, following the well-known work of Seligman (1975) on learned helplessness and depression. This time her subjects were 25 back pain sufferers and 25 matched pain-free controls. On the basis of interview and questionnaire data she concluded that universal helplessness was the norm in these patients, who saw themselves as victims of a malign fate rather than of their own personal inadequacies. The use of attribution theory might help to throw new light on the relationship between pain, activity level, and depression.

Chronic pain and depression tend to coexist. However, the majority of psychiatrists do not relish being asked to see chronic back sufferers, perhaps because their expertise has little to offer whereas the stigma of psychiatric referral is still far from banished. Sternbach (1974: 88) has suggested that the patient with a sharp and isolated peak on the Depression Scale of the MMPI may be a candidate for antidepressive medication (and hence presumably for psychiatric referral); but although such patients are by no means rare, it is not our experience that they can usually be helped in this way. Where depression – or what is often better construed as demoralization – is a rational response to depressing circumstances, it is debatable whether a pharmaceutical approach can be expected to pay dividends. Reduction of self-pity and promotion of a more positive attitude may count for more, or this at least is what lies at the heart of most behavioural re-education programmes. Behaviourists have been accused at times of a naïve philosophy, and this was certainly true of some workers in the early days of the movement. But naïvety in capable hands can be a powerful force for good, and the advantages of coaxing reluctant movers into action have been fully documented.

Finally, let us spare a thought for the patient (usually female) who has taken to her bed for weeks on end and resolutely refuses to be shifted. I have occasionally been forced to add to my mileage for this reason, and have learnt to dread such visits. One patient was a widow living alone and visited daily by an agency nurse, with strong support also from her sister and brother-in-law who lived almost on her doorstep; other patients were being attended by a sexual (though not very sexual) partner, or in two cases by ageing parents. To call on such a patient is like being received into the royal presence, be it sympathetically gracious or unashamedly cantankerous. If ever there was a case of hysteria reinforced by fond indulgence, this is it. To think in terms of gradual remobilization may be unrealistic, for the patient has often too much to lose by rising from her sick bed. Age has ranged from early twenties to late sixties, and there is no common thread apart from one who exploits and others who allow themselves to be exploited. To the casual onlooker this must seem like the end of the road, and in one unforgettable instance it has led to actual suicide. It is as if the individual has abdicated all responsibility for normal living, and is defying her next-of-kin to take drastic action. Work, leisure activities, and social life have been equally compromised, and there is no obvious way of breaking the deadlock. Counselling of the relatives is seldom rapidly effective in these cases, and marital or family therapy would be an ambitious aim. The professional worker, of whatever discipline or persuasion, may be hard put to maintain a positive approach. These are the patients most likely to cause frustration and ultimately despair in all those who are called upon to help them.

Chapter five

Pain as a distress signal

So far we have been inclined to accept the argument that to promote normal activity is often the most hopeful if not the only viable policy for managing patients with chronic but non-specific back pain. However, in so doing we must not lose sight of the very real distress which is a hallmark of persistent pain of any nature and from whatever source. This is what has to be faced by any clinician exposed time and again to the back pain sufferer. A major contribution to our understanding of the associated distress has come from Waddell (1987), whose pioneering studies in Glasgow over the past ten years or more have already been mentioned. All along he seems to have been aware of the need for inter-disciplinary collaboration in both clinical practice and research, and he too has worked closely with a clinical psychologist. Indeed we shall have occasion to draw also on the work of his colleague Main (1987), whose review of psychological interventions covers a wide spectrum.

Despite an impressive record of achievement in the conquest of disease during the twentieth century, there are many residual problems to be faced by the medical profession. Waddell has laid great stress on the meaning of 'abnormal illness behaviour' in the context of back pain. This helps to focus attention on the *owner* of the bad back, whose distress is unlikely to be relieved by a purely mechanistic approach to the vertebral column. It is largely to his insight that we owe the concept of *magnified pain presentation*, for the recognition of which he has drawn up a list of symptoms and signs (Waddell *et al*. 1980; Waddell, Bircher, *et al*. 1984; Waddell, Main, *et al*. 1984). This is a specific illustration of the more general concept of abnormal illness behaviour, which has caught the interest of psychiatrists among others (e.g. Pilowsky and Spence 1975, 1976; Pilowsky *et al*. 1977). Now some doctors are adept at seeing their patients as distressed human beings first and foremost, rather than merely as exhibitors of various bodily disturbances. This will enable them to work at a psychological level where necessary, though more often through their own laboriously acquired intuitions than as a result of anything in their clinical training. But there remain many factors – both personal and bureaucratic – that conspire to perpetuate a blinkered view of suffering humanity, and here the hospital-based specialist may be less educable than his colleagues in primary care. For if the GP's letter of referral does not usually make clear how much he already knows about the patient as a person, the specialist's response is often dictated by his traditional and narrowly interpreted terms of reference. Pressure of demand and consequent lack of opportunity for leisurely explorations are sufficient to explain the shortcomings of our overstretched outpatient services, and this is commonly acknowledged as an inescapable reality. However, it has not deterred a few enthusiasts from adapting the service to meet the patients' needs, albeit at the cost of an extended waiting list.

The *medical model*, with its simplified view of cause and effect in physical illness, has come under attack from social and behavioural scientists over the past decade or two. It may well be that chronic disorders of any kind call for a different perspective, one that seeks above all to encompass their multifactorial origin. Maintenance of good health, like any other aspect of successful living, is mediated through an untold variety of factors. We cannot reasonably expect that all such factors will be equally open to inspection; and in conceding that some individuals are inherently more vulnerable to illness than others, we may need to accept that different constitutional factors will interact with personal experience, both past and current. The study of *life events* has reached a point where, although there is broad agreement on a hierarchy of universal crises (bereavement, severe injury, sudden redundancy, and so forth), the meaning of any such event for the affected person has to be considered before its impact can be properly gauged or anticipated. This is surely part of the reason why measures for the relief of chronic pain, whether emanating from clinicians or scientists and conceived from whatever theoretical standpoint, are so hard to evaluate conclusively. What works for one person in a particular context will do nothing for another person in a different context, whilst a third person whose life is going through an altogether more problematical phase may suffer further setbacks.

Psychological approaches to the management of back pain

Over the past few years several other wide-ranging review articles have been published apart from the one by Main (1987). They have embraced biofeedback and hypnosis as well as the more popular methods of relaxation training, behavioural re-education, and cognitive therapy (Tan 1982; Turner and Chapman 1982a, 1982b; Turk and Flor 1984). All in all they afford no grounds for optimism that a major breakthrough is on the horizon, nor any reason for believing that one approach is consistently more effective than another. In this respect the newer psychological interventions are no more predictable or specific in their effects than the longer established methods of physical medicine. Indeed Flor and Turk (1984), in lamenting the paucity of controlled studies of somatic interventions, conclude that no single approach to date has proved its reliability. They suggest that some sort of interaction between physical and psychological factors may be involved in the passage to chronicity, which seems plausible enough even if not greatly illuminating. In their companion review of psychological interventions (Turk and Flor 1984) they are rueful in their criticisms of research design, whilst apparently less concerned about the relatively small numbers of patients recruited into most of the projects surveyed. Only passing reference is made to the possible contribution of well-controlled individual case studies, which in the opinion of some psychologists may hold the key to future progress. Dogged determination matched by naïve faith may have helped to launch this avalanche of recent therapeutic trials, yet had psychologists been inspired by a more realistic awareness of the many pitfalls, the long-suffering patient might have benefited more from fewer enquiries.

Significantly Waddell (1987), for all the clarity of his observations on the distress that goes with magnified pain presentation, has little to say about how it should be treated. To appreciate the reality of a patient's distress is undoubtedly the first step, and it is perhaps hardly within a surgeon's province to set about relieving it – for even if he were adept at dealing with his patients' emotional problems, he might want to protest that this was not the most appropriate use of his time and skills. Let us therefore look to his collaborator for guidance on the various options available. For his exposition, Main has drawn on nearly two hundred sources; if his conclusions as to the role of the psychologist are essentially modest, this is surely a true reflection of the present state of the art. He echoes Waddell in highlighting the possible value of stress reduction techniques and various kinds of psychotherapy 'directed not so much at the pain experience itself, but at its effects in the form of disability and invalidism' (Main 1987: 451). He goes on to plead for a switch from the traditional disease model to one incorporating the broader aspects of individual anguish in response to pain. From such a perspective any attempt at discriminating between 'organic' and 'functional' states is unhelpful, since we are unlikely to be faced with such a crude differential diagnosis once the complaint has become chronic. Nor does an emphasis on the patient's subjective experience automatically rule out physical methods of management, unless these have been tried intensively or extensively and found wanting. But Main is surely right to point out that prolonged adherence to conventional medicine *without* stopping to consider these broader aspects may be counterproductive, especially where the sufferer has been moving inexorably along a conveyor belt of opinions and recommendations in both the NHS and the private sector.

Indeed, research by the Glasgow team (Waddell, Bircher, *et al.* 1984) has demonstrated that abnormal illness behaviour is apt to be enhanced by the failure of previous conservative treatments. This important finding has been mirrored in our own clinical experience, so that we have come to see it as part of our task to dissuade some of our patients from their everlasting quest for a therapeutic holy grail. We are in complete agreement with Main when he writes:

> Failed treatment and repeatedly negative investigations maintain the patient in a passive invalid role with little expectation that he or she can influence the course of his or her pain or disability. The simple organic–functional dichotomy may have led to attributions of hypochondriasis or malingering, not only by the medical profession but also by the patient's family.
>
> (Main 1987: 452)

Possibly not the least valuable quality of the experienced clinician confronted with chronic pain is to know when to leave well alone. Doctors who directly aggravate their patients' discomfort by injudicious therapy have probably always been outnumbered by those who allow them to become slowly worse through a constant pursuit of false trails.

In reviewing specific methods of intervention by the psychologist, we shall have little to add about what has become the most popular form of behavioural re-education in the USA, namely operant training. Pioneered by Fordyce (1976) and further developed on a broader basis by other behaviourally minded psychologists (e.g. Anderson *et al.* 1977; Roberts and Reinhardt 1980; Keefe *et al.* 1981; Heinrich *et al.* 1985), it was discussed at some length in the previous chapter following a detailed clinical example in Chapter 3. It calls for the precise identification of target behaviours (pain complaints, withdrawal from activity, resort to medication, etc.) and their environmental consequences, with a view to removing or modifying the latter in such a way as to promote desired behavioural change. Despite its all-pervasive influence – which is doubtless to be understood as part of a wider trend towards behavioural medicine in clinical psychology – its effectiveness still has to be taken largely on trust. Tightly controlled studies have remained elusive, whilst successful outcome appears to be heavily dependent on the exclusion or disappearance of poorly motivated clients who would be unlikely to benefit but will nevertheless continue to seek help. Thus it may bring substantial relief from pain to the favoured few, but this is not in any case the prime objective. We shall dismiss it from further consideration here precisely because it is not explicitly designed for the relief of pain and its associated distress, unlike any of the following alternatives.

Relaxation training

People vary not only in the extent but also in the manner of their physiological reactions to stress. For example, some demonstrate increased cardiovascular activity (such as accelerated heart rate), others enhanced galvanic skin response, and others again amplified muscle activity. The aim of stress reduction techniques is therefore to redress the presumptive autonomic imbalance.

Chronic back pain may give rise to localized muscular tension of a kind that persists long after the original injury has healed, with the result that a pain–tension cycle will become firmly established. The ensuing anxiety can only compound the problem, and by reducing the patient's anxiety one may hope to provide some degree of control over the pain. Hence progressive muscular relaxation, as practised by other professions besides clinical psychology, is intended initially as a means of countering anxiety and only secondarily as a remedy for pain. A variety of techniques have been tried, most of which involve systematic tensing and relaxing of different muscle groups throughout the body. Whilst the role of the therapist is not to be underestimated, some patients have learnt to achieve freedom from tension through self-instruction (so-called autogenic training).

It is perhaps hardly surprising that this approach to the management of chronic pain syndromes has proved most effective with tension headaches (Tasto and Hinkle 1973) and migraine (Hay and Madders 1971). The fact that people complain of headache rather than head pain is surely in itself significant; clinical experience would suggest, albeit in the absence of direct evidence, that headache patients as compared with back pain sufferers are often more ready to acknowledge the role of tension in their condition. Whether stress is a more powerful contributory factor in the case of headache is open to debate, but *a priori* there is no particular reason why it should be. However, at a practical level it may be easier to persuade the individual with an incapacitating headache to engage in relaxation training if the immediate effect is beneficial, whereas it may even be aversive in the case of severe back pain. Yet this does not detract from the argument for introducing relaxation classes into any rehabilitation programme for chronic back pain sufferers, as recently at the Wolfson Centre where they have proved acceptable to most patients taking part.

There has been little attempt to test the specific value of relaxation for chronic back pain, since it is normally offered as one element of a composite treatment programme. In the study by Keefe *et al.* (1981), for instance, it was combined with biofeedback and educational advice, which made it impossible to determine how much it had contributed to the overall success of the regime. In contrast, Sanders (1983) was able by means of a balanced design to show that it played a more important part than either assertion training, social reinforcement for increased activity, or

a functional pain-behaviour analysis; whilst a controlled comparison of group relaxation and cognitive-behavioural therapy (Turner
1982) indicated that both treatment groups fared better on various
outcome measures than patients who remained on a waiting list.
However, one cannot be too optimistic about the prospect of
neatly disentangling the influences of diverse remedial measures
upon any non-specific complaint such as back pain. If what is
required above all else is a *therapeutic milieu* in which different
treatments can be allowed to interact with more powerful effect
than would be expected of any single treatment in isolation, then
some of the reported experimental work might be called into
question even on ethical grounds.

Hypnosis

As a technique that can be deployed in a variety of contexts,
remedial and otherwise, hypnosis has both a chequered history
and a lasting mystical aura. It was used by surgeons in the days
before the discovery of inhalant anaesthetics; it was used by Freud
to remove troublesome symptoms, until he discovered its
seductive properties with hysterical young women; it continues to
be used as a means of pain control in such disparate fields as
dentistry and childbirth; and it has enabled showmen to hold a
theatre audience with riveting demonstrations of such intriguing
phenomena as age regression (eliciting childlike behaviour) and
post-hypnotic suggestion (getting the subject to perform quasi-
automatic actions after emerging from a trance). Yet despite its
multifarious applications there are relatively few clinicians who
hold it in high esteem as a therapeutic tool. On the whole it could
be said to have inspired more laboratory-based experimental work
– mainly designed to elucidate its *modus operandi* – than remedial
action.

In some ways it could be regarded as lying along a continuum
from relaxation, which can be used to explore an individual's
readiness to be hypnotized. Only a small minority (say 10 per
cent) are totally resistant, but an equally small minority can be
led into a deep trance with ease. It is hard to predict who will
respond well, but it does not take long to find out. Given the
necessary self-confidence, most experienced clinicians could
acquire a modicum of skill. Hypnotic control over pain can be

achieved (in theory) by a number of different means, including direct suggestion of analgesia, replacing a painful sensation with a less painful one, and shifting the locus of pain either to another area of the body or right outside it. It is unfortunate that many of the more impressive demonstrations of pain reduction have been enacted on healthy volunteers submitting to experimentally induced pain rather than on involuntary sufferers (Hilgard and Hilgard 1986).

Careful evaluations of hypnosis in the management of back pain have been few and far between. In choosing to work with patients who had a history of lumbar surgery Crasilneck (1979) was unlikely to be making his task any easier, although all but 4 of his 24 patients proved susceptible to hypnosis. Moreover considerable pain relief was reported by 16 subjects during the first four sessions, with an estimated overall reduction of 70 per cent after six sessions. In the absence of follow-up enquiry or an appropriate control group this short-term response cannot be regarded as more than suggestive. In another small-scale enquiry (n = 17) McCauley *et al.* (1983) found that self-hypnosis and relaxation were equally effective as taught to out-patients over eight weekly sessions; the drop-out rate was higher in the relaxation group, but the hypnosis group called for a heavier investment of professional skills. The authors end by conceding quite serious limitations in the design of their study, and we are still a long way from knowing any of the factors that might favour one approach over the other.

Biofeedback

A more technically sophisticated form of stress reduction is biofeedback, in which physiological events – typically muscular contraction in this context – are electronically monitored and the information is displayed either visually or aurally in order to bring normally unconscious processes within voluntary control. On the assumption that some physiological aberration may have been adding to the severity of the pain, patients have an opportunity to modify their pain experience by exerting control over their hidden bodily processes. As with relaxation training, biofeedback has been systematically evaluated primarily in relation to headache, for which it has been found comparably effective but generally no more so (Silver and Blanchard 1978). However, it emerged as a probably beneficial influence in the management of rheumatic back pain (Flor *et al*. 1983). In view of the more elaborate technology demanded by biofeedback many clinicians will continue to prefer the simpler of the two methods. Turk, Meichenbaum and Berman (1979), on the evidence available to them, urged caution in promoting the use of biofeedback, and similar reservations were expressed more recently by Melzack and Wall (1988). However, there will always be some patients who respond to the mystique of electronic apparatus, which may indeed give them a sense of mastery over their pain.

Cognitive therapy

In contrast to any of the foregoing approaches, cognitive methods of pain control seek their effect through altering the sufferer's attitudes and expectations. There are introverts who habitually pay close attention to their inner thoughts and feelings, having perhaps never learned to ignore minor discomfort; and perfectionists who are hoist with the petard of their own unrealistically high expectations of bodily integrity, being unable to tolerate even minor departures from an ideal state. These are overlapping classes, but there are many other individuals whose pain experience appears to be out of all proportion to their physical problems. Procedures for counteracting some of these self-defeating tendencies have been thoroughly documented by Turk *et al*. (1983), although convincing studies of their efficacy are still awaited. Whilst there can be no denying the relevance of attitudinal factors in pain experience, I have yet to be persuaded that this particular theoretical stance is ever likely to revolutionize the treatment of psychological disorders. But if adaptability means shaping one's own responses to accommodate life's negative experiences, there is no reason in theory why part of this capacity for survival could not be taught. Such has always been a fundamental aim of counselling and psychotherapy, to be considered in the next section.

If the manner in which events are appraised has a critical bearing on emotional experiences, whether positive or negative, then it ought to be possible to help an individual to cope with pain by appropriate indoctrination. This has been attempted in relation to elective surgery, as for example by providing information and advice on coping strategies prior to hysterectomy (Ridgeway and Mathews 1982). Preparing someone for an impending ordeal of this kind is obviously quite a different matter from helping them to cope with chronic pain of unknown origin; and even with surgical patients the results of cognitive preparation are seldom dramatic. Thus not all such patients are anxious for information, and people vary in their habitual styles of coping with threat (Wallace 1984). All the same, one might hope that there are some lessons to be learned from the management of actual and anticipated pain in hospital, and this is currently a growth area for the experimentally minded clinical psychologist. If Main's review of cognitive therapy is disappointing in terms of hard findings, this is again partly due to an apparent preference among researchers for combining it with other approaches to pain management.

Meanwhile there have been a few hopeful straws in the wind. Cognitive factors appeared to be playing some part in a self-management programme for reducing medication in chronic back pain sufferers (Alperson et al. 1984), while several other clinical studies have attested to the possible influence of such factors on the outcome of treatment. In an interesting project by Large (1985), using personal construct theory to measure self-dissatisfaction and electromyographic feedback as the experimental intervention, it was reported that virtually all participants in an out-patient pain management programme saw themselves as less seriously ill at the end of it even if no significant improvements were achieved in their ratings of either pain or mood state. Any induced modification of attitude to illness, provided that it is reinforced rather than counteracted by subsequent experience, may open the way to better control over pain.

As well as seeking to alter cognitive appraisal of the situation, coping strategies may also (or instead) be aimed at diverting attention from the pain (Turk et al. 1983). Sufferers may be urged to focus on a mental image incompatible with pain, such as musical rapture or sexual arousal; or they may be encouraged to reinterpret their pain as a different kind of sensation, such as numbness. These and various other measures may be employed in an effort to reduce anxiety and subacute pain, and hopefully also to persuade the patient that he or she rather than the therapist has prime responsibility for effective management of chronic pain. If only some sense of control can be passed to the sufferer, it may help to alleviate the element of learnt helplessness that is so destructive in the long run. Counteracting a sense of helplessness was one of three helpful strategies identified by Rosenstiel and Keefe (1983) in their study of sixty-one chronic back patients, the other two being cognitive coping/suppression and diverting attention, especially by prayer. An attractive feature of cognitive therapy is its scope for creative imagination and flexibility, but this is probably also a major drawback when it comes to validating its claims. Like the treatments inspired by personal construct theory (which was mentioned briefly above), it is idiosyncratic rather than normative, giving rise to a wide range of individual variation and thereby largely stultifying all attempt at predicting therapeutic response by means of controlled intergroup comparisons.

Finally, it is perhaps worth noting – even if it ought to be self-evident – that cognitive therapy is more accurately conceived as cognitive-behavioural therapy. If its overriding objective is to promote better coping skills, then its effects are ultimately best judged in terms of actual behaviour. Attitudes may be important as a mediating variable, but if the nature and level of the sufferer's daily activities remain unchanged it is doubtful how much if anything has been gained.

Counselling and psychotherapy

The early days of the behaviour therapy movement were characterized by a search for methods of intervention that would be relatively independent of the personal qualities of the therapist. If hopes and expectations of this kind were realistic then it ought to be possible to make extensive use of tape-recorded instructions and other time-saving measures, with resultant gains in cost-effectiveness and availability. Clinical experience has confirmed that there is indeed plenty of scope for self-instruction, self-monitoring, and the use of audiovisual aids, notably in relaxation training. However, it is fair to suggest that in the end there is no substitute for skilled individual handling of the patient, whether in establishing rapport at the outset and securing maximum co-operation, or in monitoring the progress of treatment. With the wisdom of hindsight it is perhaps hard to imagine how it would ever be possible or desirable to dispense with the virtuoso skills of the highly trained clinician, of whatever persuasion. But it is above all in the area of counselling and psychotherapy that a huge gulf becomes apparent between the ordinarily competent and the outstandingly gifted. Practitioners among the helping professions vary as much as in any other calling, and some patients may remain in pain simply because they have never been lucky enough to meet a sufficiently skilled therapist.

But is there anything in the notion that psychosomatic patients are too well defended against their emotions to make good candidates for psychotherapy, even at the most superficial level? Sifneos (1973) has argued that such patients are more likely to deteriorate in response to any attempt at in-depth interpretation of their symptoms, and Karasu (1979) was equally pessimistic about the value of a psychodynamic approach to the 'medically ill'. This negative evaluation of psychotherapy in the context of ostensibly physical illness has become firmly entrenched, so that the contemporary literature on psychological interventions has little to say about it. Reductive – as opposed to merely supportive – psychotherapy has tended to be favoured for patients who display a measure of insight into their emotional problems without taking refuge in bodily symptoms. Prima facie it has to be recognized that chronic pain patients are scarcely noted for their capacity to think psychologically. That chronic back sufferers are notably *deficient* in this capacity is a possibility that cannot be ruled out.

In the course of assessing several hundred pain patients, I have tried to remain alert to the possibility of offering help of this nature to carefully selected patients. Regrettably it must be said that opportunities have been limited, and a more pragmatic approach to the management of pain has usually had to suffice. Many patients might stand to gain from detailed information on their pain problem and advice on how its worst effects could be mitigated; few are looking for guidance on what has conspired to make them the kind of person they are, or for enlightenment as to the basis of their long-term maladaptive responses to living. After all, it has always been painful to face the truth about oneself. Many of us spend much of our time in flight from self-awareness, or in constructing a false picture of ourselves as a protection against coming to terms with what lies behind the uneasy façade. And to a certain extent chronic bodily pain can serve as a metaphor for the pain of living. As Menges (1981: 95) has observed, 'One could say that it is not the pain that is unbearable but life without that pain.' From this perspective it may become easier to understand why some patients are more than a little reluctant to give up their pain, having nothing more rewarding to put in its place. These are the patients who could be regarded as most in need of psychotherapy but at the same time most strongly fortified against its invasion of the self. A compelling example of this sad state of affairs will be given in the next chapter, which will also address the question of group therapy. Meanwhile I shall comment briefly on two issues not so far considered explicitly: the concept of the multidisciplinary pain programme, and the need to develop more satisfactory criteria of outcome.

The multidisciplinary approach

In concluding his review of psychological interventions with a brief survey of multidisciplinary pain programmes, Main (1987) has drawn almost exclusively on the American literature of the past ten years. Britain and Australia have been slow to catch up with this trend, although a number of British psychologists besides Main have made it their business to familiarize themselves with the transatlantic scene. Plainly our own health care system does not lend itself so readily to pain clinics of this type, which are expensive to run, whilst an acute shortage of clinical psychologists might well be another factor. At the time of writing only the pain relief unit at Walton Hospital in Liverpool has become nationally known for offering a service of this nature; and if indeed it is virtually a unique service in this country then it must be heavily oversubscribed.

Pain clinics in the USA vary widely in their administration, clientele, treatment philosophy, and range of methods employed. Back sufferers account for a substantial minority of some groups and a clear majority of others. Some programmes are non-residential, others admit for a brief period (typically about three weeks). A fair number offer a sensible combination of physical and psychological methods of rehabilitation, in that mobility and tolerance of discomfort can be extended through graded exercises, whilst attitudes and expectations can be modified through professionally led discussion groups. Stress reduction techniques as described earlier are in regular use. Most patients are followed up for long enough at least to assess the immediate impact of the regime, and an overview of the better established pain units has been available for some years (Aronoff *et al.* 1983). This movement towards comprehensive management of chronic pain, with all its attendant distress and disability, is to be welcomed as a clinical enterprise if not also as an exercise in controlled research.

Turning to the question of outcome, it is hard to envisage any universally acceptable criteria. The patients arrive at different stages of their 'pain career', with widely varying employment histories and all manner of current living arrangements. And just as their response to the programme is almost infinitely variable, so they will elicit a variety of responses from staff members and fellow sufferers. There is simply no way of contriving a standard yardstick whereby to evaluate a standard patient undergoing a standardized regime. Moreover, a short spell of residential treatment, for all its advantages in terms of respite from family stress coinciding with a degree of control over immediate experience, is but a drop in the ocean of daily living unless it can trigger a major reorganization of the patient's whole *modus vivendi*. Sometimes a few weeks away from normal routine for whatever reason can serve as a crucial turning point in a person's life, but the odds are heavily against it. In reality most pain patients return to their all too familiar scene. This observation, for which no originality is claimed, can be illustrated with findings from a carefully conducted study of 151 back pain sufferers in Helsinki (Mellin *et al.* 1984). All were men aged 54–63 with a history of interference with daily activities in the absence of other incapacitating long-term illness. Some 60 per cent underwent three weeks' formal rehabilitation at a spa, the rest being managed as out-patients for a similar period. When the two groups were followed up at set intervals after discharge and compared on measurements of spinal function as well as a back pain index derived from questionnaire responses, the effects of the two treatments were much the same. In itself this is no cause for dismay, for clearly there is no royal road to improvement; but it has to be disappointing that the therapeutic effects began to wear off after six months on average and had disappeared almost completely within a year.

Even so, the short-term gains demonstrated in this and many other studies are not to be underestimated. After a long period in the wilderness it is not unreasonable to attribute beneficial changes to an intensive therapeutic regime rather than to spontaneous remission. What would lead to significant advances in pain management is a better understanding of predictive factors. Those most frequently considered – such as age, social status, duration of disability – are not the most subtly influential. Personality tests such as the MMPI, cumbersome though still ubiquitous in the USA, are moderately effective in screening out the doubtful starter (Humphrey 1980). But we need also to be able to recognize the good bet, and here we have a long way to go. That a global measure of distress, the Derogatis Brief Symptom Inventory (Derogatis and Spencer 1982), predicted outcome better than pre-existing intensity of pain was an encouraging feature of a preliminary report by Wharton *et al.* (1984). If this sort of finding could be widely replicated it would reinforce the theme of this chapter, which is that patients would be more effectively managed if the spotlight was switched from pain as such to the overall level of distress. For whilst distress is no less subjective than pain, it is more amenable to a variety of well-tried measuring instruments.

Coping with distress

When confronted with distress on a grand scale even the seasoned clinician can readily be made to feel uncomfortable. Possibly this is harder still for the paramedical worker, whose training may be less geared to the acceptance of human suffering as a reality; be that as it may, there will always be some patients with a highly developed capacity for wreaking havoc on the multidisciplinary team. How are such patients to be managed? Obviously there is no easy answer to this question, but let us first consider how often distress is unmistakably declared at a special back pain clinic.

If the MMPI profile can be accepted as an overall measure of distress, whatever its diagnostic limitations, then our clientele divide more or less equally into three groups: the non-distressed (whose overt behaviour may nevertheless belie their normal profile), the severely distressed, and an intermediate group with borderline features. Of some two hundred patients referred for independent psychological assessment over the past four years, rather more than half were given a semi-structured interview as well as completing the MMPI and the two pencil-and-paper questionnaires described in the previous chapter. Rapid inspection of the psychological reports led to the immediate identification of six women and two men as severely distressed at their first attendance. All were seen again at least once and most several times, giving ample opportunity to confirm initial impressions. A third man was seen on a home visit without being tested, but in view of his presenting symptoms and psychiatric history (which began with two suicide attempts as an adolescent) he can confidently be assigned to the severely distressed group.[1] These nine patients, representing almost 5 per cent of my case-load over this period, ranged in age from 27 to 57, but most were in their thirties or forties. Six were married and the other three were cohabiting; however, conspicuous problems emerged in most of these relationships. The only married man, who was a self-employed builder, claimed that his marriage had remained unimpaired by the trauma of losing the first daughter from sudden illness two years before and having to cope with severe mental handicap in the second one. (The third daughter was barely a toddler, and his wife appeared only for the first interview – there was illness in the family to keep her from the second interview, whilst on the most recent occasion she had been admitted to hospital with hypertension of pregnancy.) Of the two cohabiting men one was a homosexual in a stable but somewhat uneasy partnership, the other had formed a relationship with a nurse at the psychiatric unit where he had been treated only a few months earlier. Socially and occupationally these patients came from all walks of life.

The selection of these cases was made on the basis of vivid recollection and without detailed reference to the MMPI record, which was found to be borderline or within normal limits for three women. The prevalence of overt marital problems in this small group was at variance with the picture of enduring stability conveyed by most of our patients, as documented in Chapter 3 (see Humphrey and Jones 1987). It is perhaps not unreasonable to suppose that distress in a married woman with chronic pain is in some way inversely proportional to the quality of emotional support from her partner, but this would be hard to measure. At all events there were no manifestly 'golden' husbands hovering around these unhappy creatures. Probably the most seriously distressed of all was married to a homosexual estate agent, who had plainly never been equal to her erotic needs and so had more than once driven her into the arms of another man. Though deeply wounded by her infidelity he had tolerated it over the years, until the misfortune of aggravating a long-standing lumbar weakness in a fall had deprived her of other pleasures besides those of the bed. There was little enough scope for marital therapy in such a doomed relationship, and it might not be too fanciful to look upon the pain as a forlorn attempt to expiate her guilt feelings. When last seen the couple were gloomily on the verge of retiring to a rural area, where they would be virtually alone with their problems.

Three husbands in this small group had been unfaithful to their wives who had thought about leaving them, although the youngest wife was effectively tied by her children. The two older women would to all intents and purposes have relished their freedom, but somehow lacked the courage to make a clean break. In such circumstances it would be sanguine to hope for a dramatic response to specific methods of pain management, whereas abrupt resolution of the conflict might lead to a spontaneous remission. In any case resources for helping these and other patients at a psychological level have always been heavily stretched, since individual therapy is so time-consuming. The possibility of group therapy for married couples has recently been explored, but this would presumably have more to offer where the patient was in a viable relationship.

Anyone on the lookout for pain as a distress signal would have no difficulty in recognizing it, but usually it is much easier to recognize than to treat. It is also easier to write about than to manage effectively, which is why so few therapists write and so few writers engage in therapy. Setting out to discover whether one approach is superior to another can be viewed as an even greater challenge. Regrettably it is hard to avoid the impression that many of the studies reviewed in this chapter are simplistic, in the sense that their authors display little or no sign of having faced up to the complexity of pain as a therapeutic target. Of course, not all sufferers are as hard to help as the middle-aged woman who clings desperately to a failed marriage. However, the fact that so many chronic pain patients are middle-aged is not really in their favour. Many of them have a long history, and some may see themselves as facing a bleak future.

Life in mid-marriage and mid-career may have become a little smoother in some respects, with earlier crises surmounted and children beginning to leave home. But there is still a long way to go for most, with declining energies to cope with the degenerative disorders of the ageing process. So the future can be daunting even without a pain problem, as traffic multiplies, public services steadily deteriorate, and options for living begin to narrow. How can the person with a bad back hope to keep going amid all these frustrations? Some of the chronic patients who seek help could be forgiven for wanting to curl up and die, but they soldier on. Miraculously not all have entirely lost heart.

Chapter six

The need for self-help

As chronic back pain is such a mysterious ailment we cannot be surprised that treatment is largely empirical. Almost nothing can be stated with confidence about the relative efficacy of alternative methods, although we can be sure that almost anything has been known to bring relief to some sufferers some of the time. Even such a simple and apparently innocuous remedy as complete bed rest has to be viewed with caution, at least in the absence of manifest neurological impairment. For when more than two hundred patients presenting with 'mechanical' low back pain were recruited into a randomized trial to compare the benefits of two days versus seven days of bed rest, no differences in outcome could be demonstrated (Deyo *et al.* 1986). Exclusion of the less compliant patients from the seven-day group had no effect on the result, and the authors were obviously well aware of the benefit to society of restricting time off work to an absolute minimum. If time-honoured physical remedies are of unproven value – indeed retiring to bed, however briefly, may even hold up the recovery process for some people – why should we expect clear-cut answers from a comparison of the newer psychological therapies?

Perhaps the time has come, belatedly as some would argue, to pay more attention to the advantages of self-help in overcoming the worst effects of chronic pain. In their recent guidebook written from such a perspective Broome and Jellicoe are admirably succinct, even if the reader is asked to take a lot on trust. They start by declaring that 'one fact stands out above all others: the most effective changes come about when people begin to solve their problems for themselves' (Broome and Jellicoe 1987: vii). Doubtless this conviction stems from clinical experience rather than from scientific enquiry, yet it emerges just as strongly from the more closely reasoned text of Turk, Meichenbaum, and Genest. In explaining how they seek to involve their clients, these authors suggest that the therapist should lose no time in emphasizing the need for active participation:

> You have been to several doctors and clinics before you came here, so when you arrived this morning you probably had some idea of what to expect. At the same time you might have been wondering whether we would do anything differently here, perhaps hoping that finally something could be done to help. . . .
>
> Here we don't do things to you or give you *things* to change your pain. What we will be doing is helping you to use the resources *you* have to affect your pain. Now, you may think you have already tried everything, done everything you can to help yourself and I know that you do indeed want to reduce your pain and do what you can for yourself. What we are going to look for is resources that you may not be aware of and ways of using your abilities in a different manner.
>
> (Turk *et al.* 1983: 248)

In view of the refractory nature of the handicap, especially where the pain originates from the lumbar spine, remarkably few investigators have gone on record as attempting to pinpoint the characteristics of those who respond poorly to formal rehabilitation programmes. An exploratory study was undertaken by Painter *et al.* (1980), who used a postal questionnaire to identify the 25 most and 25 least successful attenders at a pain centre in terms of their status a year or so after discharge. Disability compensation, depression, and a passive-dependent stance were notable features of the least successful group, who had apparently made little effort to improve their social situation. The authors estimate that overall about one patient in four, from a total of 145 who returned the questionnaire, had failed to capitalize on their temporary improvement at the centre, so far as residual pain and functional limitations were concerned. They conclude that attitudinal factors were undoubtedly implicated, although unfortunately these could not be reliably identified at the time of attendance. Further evidence as to the nature of such factors could surely point the way to more effective management of chronic pain. Either a means must be found to induce a more positive attitude in those less inclined towards active participation, or they must be excluded from rehabilitation programmes in favour of others who could be expected to take full advantage of the opportunity for self-help.

In selecting patients for referral to the Wolfson Centre we have sometimes departed from this principle, but only because the first week of the three-to-four week programme serves as a preliminary trial. If at the end of this period a patient is deemed unsuitable for the graded series of activities, then he or she is discharged at this stage with an appropriate letter to the referring agent. Thus in a sense there is nothing to be lost by sending a few potential candidates whose strength of commitment is uncertain, since a more informed decision can usually be reached in the course of five working days. Even so, it has become our invariable practice to stress the vital importance of self-help, especially where there is more than a hint of passivity in the patient's approach to previous interventions. Sometimes we leave it to the patient to contact the clinic after further consideration of the offer. It is perhaps worth harking back here to our earlier distinction between *pacers* and *recliners*, the latter being those whose apprehensive avoidance of activity for fear of aggravating their pain may in extreme cases have virtually brought them to a standstill. It may be asking too much of even the most experienced and dedicated rehabilitation staff to galvanize such reluctant movers into action, but some unexpectedly good results have been achieved from time to time.

Turk and his colleagues have written extensively about the central role of the 'therapeutic alliance' in pain management. They criticize other therapists (albeit not by name) for taking insufficient trouble over the introductory phase of a treatment programme, which is the time to spell out the rationale in considerable detail and to enlist the client's wholehearted collaboration. If this is not done there can be no cause for complaint if the outcome is no more satisfactory than in the case of orthodox medical procedures to which he or she has passively consented in the past. Almost half of their 1983 monograph is devoted to a blow-by-blow account of their cognitive-behavioural methods, and in the opening chapter of this section they are at their most persuasive. Their theme here is compliance and resistance, and it is to this supremely relevant consideration that we shall turn next.

Communication and compliance

The teaching of the behavioural sciences (notably psychology and sociology) to medical students over the past two decades has been inevitably selective, but an informal survey I made of course content in the London medical schools has shown that communication and compliance have become a *sine qua non*. Whatever else may get left out, this composite theme is assured of a hearing. This *should* mean that tomorrow's doctors – and a good few of today's – no longer take for granted their effectiveness as communicators. Meanwhile, reports continue to appear in the literature of dissatisfied patients, not only those who have failed to improve but even more conspicuously those who claim that they were given no idea what to expect of their treatment. In view of its empirical quality there is no reason for expecting the management of back pain to be exempt from such criticisms, of which two recent examples must suffice.

From a study in Texas of 140 patients with 'mechanical' low back pain, Deyo and Diehl (1986) found that the most frequently cited source of dissatisfaction was failure to receive an adequate explanation of the problem. Discussion of symptoms, aetiology, and prognosis was left to the discretion of junior hospital staff; and as there was no tape-recording of these conversations, the true quality of the explanations proffered could not be assessed. However, the authors could find no evidence that the more dissatisfied patients were overdemanding, at least on the basis of their initial expectations elicited in a standardized interview or their self-rated improvement over the next three weeks. If Barsky (1981) is correct in suggesting that what patients often seek from physicians is primarily information, and possibly also reassurance that their disease is not serious or likely to get worse, then explanation of symptoms may go a long way towards meeting their immediate needs. Whilst careful repetition may be needed to ensure that the explanation is accurately received, it may take longer still for a doctor to communicate vague ideas in a muddled fashion.

A study of fifty patients attending a rheumatological back pain clinic in outer London came to similar conclusions about the value of clear communication, although diagnostic issues were less prominent. Fitzpatrick *et al*. (1987) interviewed these patients at home prior to their first attendance, but relied on postal questionnaires to assess level of satisfaction three months later. Apart from physiotherapy, which on the whole was not well received, dissatisfaction was focused largely on the doctor's inadequacy when it came to discussing current anxieties or future prospects. In contrast to the Texan group, of whom 70 per cent had acute pain of less than two weeks' duration, the London out-patients were biased towards chronicity with a mean duration of more than twelve months for the present episode and more than six years since the original onset. The possibility that dissatisfaction with medical care increases over time cannot be examined on account of gross differences of population and method between the two studies, but it is only to be expected that patients would voice different concerns at different stages of their disorder.

Whether the quality of the doctor's explanation as conveyed to the patient has any bearing on the passage to chronicity of pain complaint is a question that cannot be answered either. If the message is clearer for prognosis (favourable) than for diagnosis (uncertain), this may be perfectly acceptable in the earlier stages, but if the trouble persists the patient is unlikely to remain satisfied for long. Of particular interest is the patient's attitude to psychological interpretations, which has provoked more comment than systematic enquiry. Sternbach and Rusk (1973) observed that pain patients as a class were disposed to reject psychological explanations of their symptoms, so that mental health workers were seen as threatening to their dignity and self-esteem. Such resistance to the reinterpretation of their pain experience in non-physical terms may not be altogether unrealistic, in that patients with an ambiguous diagnosis are apt to be regarded by health care workers as less genuine in their pain complaints (Gillmore and Hill 1981). Waddell's concept of magnified pain presentation will be recalled in this connection; and whilst he has never sought to deny the reality of the patient's distress, this has never provided such a convincing entrée into the world of physical medicine.

Satisfaction and compliance are theoretically independent aspects of a medical consultation, yet in practice they are interwoven. The baffled or frustrated patient is unlikely to leave the doctor's surgery or out-patient clinic feeling happy about the transaction; and in the event of failure to understand what was said he (or probably more often she) will neither retain the message nor feel as strongly disposed to act on any advice given. The question of compliance has been comprehensively reviewed with reference to diverse aspects of health care such as weight reduction, medication, exercise, and other modifications of lifestyle (Dunbar 1980; Ley 1982). It is a sad but indisputable fact of human nature that people are so resistant to changing their habits, which means that more than crystal-clear communication is needed to induce behavioural change.

Dunbar (1980) has produced a sorry catalogue of misdemeanours in this context. Missed appointments were recorded for 20–50 per cent of patients, errors in use of medicines for 20–80 per cent, and premature discontinuation in 25–60 per cent according to the findings of various studies in the USA. Similarly, a clear majority of participants in programmes for controlling obesity or heavy smoking have been found to relapse or withdraw within six months or so. British experience has been no different (Ley 1982). It may have been Freud who first gave pride of place to resistance as something that had to be circumvented by the therapist before therapy could proceed, but plainly one does not have to be laid out on a psychoanalytic couch in order to display it. Much as we may insist on telling ourselves that we are determined to give up a noxious activity or take up one that is calculated to improve our health, what we actually find ourselves doing is quite another matter. Self-deception has always been endemic among those seeking to overcome their major weaknesses – or, as Oscar Wilde more memorably expressed it, 'The road to hell is paved with good intentions.'

Failure to comply with medical advice can have serious consequences. Such is not always the case and indeed the contrary may sometimes be true – witness current concern over widespread addiction to the benzodiazepines, prescribed in their millions for the relief of quite ordinary anxieties or states of tension (and thus ironically described as 'mother's little helpers'). Doctors too can be harassed almost beyond endurance, until they are led into prescribing uncritically without thought for either the underlying malaise or the undesirable after-effects. A patient's opposition to recommended procedures ought not to be seen as 'vaguely sinful' if there is any chance that it could be construed as a healthy reaction (Davidson 1976: 248). Objections of this kind can be ruled out where the advantages of strict compliance should be self-evident. When patients undergoing treatment for glaucoma were warned that they would go blind unless they could get into the habit of instilling their eye drops three times a day, departures from the regimen were reported by more than half of the group (Vincent 1971). Even those who were already legally blind in one eye were not significantly more compliant than those who retained useful vision in both eyes (59 versus 41 per cent). What on earth can be done to counteract this seemingly casual approach to prevention? Pain patients too can be their own worst enemies through failing to take sensible instructions to heart.

At our weekly clinic no opportunity is lost to explain to patients how they can hope to keep their pain within manageable bounds, as by wearing a corset, shedding a few surplus pounds (or stones), avoiding activities that have been found to make it worse, and taking particular care over lifting, seating arrangements, and other traps for the unwary. These are lessons that the 'back school' at the Wolfson Centre is designed to reinforce. However, most patients who have been in pain for months if not years are already only too well aware of the need to live within their limitations. They have been advised by other health care workers in the past, or they have discovered for themselves. But aside from the twin problems of conflicting views among the helping professions and divergent interpretations on the patient's part, we are up against the realities of daily life. It is unrealistic to expect anyone to perform every single task or chosen activity in a calculated manner from dawn till dusk; constant vigilance may be the patient's best protection against chronic pain, but there is always the unguarded moment. Hence the familiar story of a patient surviving recognizable hazards, only to succumb to the most seemingly trivial provocation – the unheralded sneeze, the half-conscious reaching for the alarm clock, or the instinctive response to an upset toddler. Self-discipline may go a long way towards warding off the feared relapse, but it ranks as a necessary rather than as a sufficient condition.

Here the chronic pain victim is in much the same position as the amateur musician who knows only too well how he ought to be practising his favourite pieces for best results, yet is for ever falling into the trap of speeding up over the easier passages. This increased tempo is too fast for the harder passages, which must be played slowly if they are to be note-perfect. It requires unflagging self-discipline to maintain a consistently slow tempo throughout, and this is a mark of professionalism. Most back pain sufferers are amateurs at heart when it comes to the detailed mechanics of everyday living. How then can they be helped to become more professional, which is essentially what compliance is all about? Only by constant persuasion during the time that they are expected to benefit from discreet supervision by health care workers. Unless and until they are ready to 'go it alone' by taking full responsibility for their own well-being, they cannot be regarded as on the road to recovery. Such a statement of the philosophy of self-help may give the impression of being unduly severe, and it is not meant to imply any disparagement of the medical or allied professions. Further consultation may be perfectly justified in the event of any new problems emerging, but almost anything is better than the compulsive search for new remedies when the old problem persists.

Before turning to the question of group support as an adjunct to self-help, let us illustrate the difficulties that can arise for the individual who resolutely refuses to acknowledge the role of self-help in adaptation to chronic back pain.

An unmarried woman of 33 was readmitted to the Wolfson Centre for a further brief course of rehabilitation. Her first episode of back pain was some time previously, but it had recurred more recently within the context of an emotional crisis and had persisted with only minor fluctuations over the past three years.

At the age of 17 she had fallen madly in love with a cousin who lived abroad. She herself is personable enough, but she portrayed him in conventionally glowing terms as not only tall, dark, and handsome, but a paragon of physical fitness, as might be expected of an ex-paratrooper. Their relationship over the years could be described as volatile, and it was doubtful whether at any time they had arrived at an understanding that sooner or later they would marry. However, she was never one to abandon hope, and it was during a visit to her cousin's home that she became incapacitated by a sudden recrudescence of her pain. Her aunt, who had never approved of the relationship, lost no time in despatching her back to England with her future still unresolved (in her own mind, that is – the cousin's viewpoint remains unknown).

Prior to this unfortunate visit she had been working as a creative writer, apparently with at least a modicum of success. On returning home to live with her widowed mother she had remained quite unable to contemplate any form of work until a few months after her initial spell of rehabilitation, when almost on impulse she applied for an unusual post as a part-time writer in residence at a hospital some distance from where her mother lived. She was not offered the post, which in retrospect she thought would have been well beyond her physical resources anyway.

When last seen after an interval of six months or more she was still politely sceptical in response to the suggestion that she should boldly take charge of her life – belatedly as it seemed to me – rather than continue in the almost certainly mistaken conviction that her only hope was to ease herself back to normal living through a series of infinitesimally gradual stages. Although professing herself eager to resume work, she let slip in conversation that her most pressing need was to be well enough to resume contact with her cousin.

It might be supposed that if it was her destiny to marry him she would have done so long ago, but she was evidently loth to face the future on this basis. As it happened she was halfway through the first draft of an autobiographical novel, but she was equally resistant to the advice that she should give priority to finishing this in the hope that it might promote some insight and clarify her options for living. To do so she would need to increase her sitting tolerance day by day and week by week until she could manage an hour or two at her typewriter without interruption (it being much harder to compose in short snatches). As yet she had found it all too easy to persuade herself that the time was not ripe for this.

By any standards this was a striking example of back pain complicated by emotional problems, and she had to press hard to be readmitted so soon after her initial spell. Previously she had been seen by other specialists, and a neurologist whom she had consulted privately appeared utterly perplexed by her condition (which nevertheless had seemed to respond well to a brief period of physiotherapy as an in-patient). It would appear that nobody had ever thought to enquire into the psychological significance of her symptoms, although there were obvious signs that her life was not quite as it should be. Any undue emphasis on the physical aspects of her rehabilitation was in danger of becoming counterproductive; indeed it could be argued that vital opportunities had already been missed.

Compliance with the dictates of clinical management – be it medical or psychological – presupposes that a number of conditions are being met if the patient is to have a reasonable chance of recovering or at least improving. First, there must be plausible grounds for believing that a particular treatment or style of management is appropriate for a particular individual in the light of all the known facts. This is often no easy matter to decide where the sufferer is in a complex situation, which may have evolved over many years as in the case just quoted. Second, the plan of action must be conveyed to all concerned in the clearest possible terms, with ample opportunity to raise queries or objections to what is being proposed. Third, the patient must accept an element of accountability to a designated key worker, at any rate until there is sufficient evidence that the necessary self-control has been established. Doubtless other conditions could readily be specified, but by now it should be abundantly clear that self-help is neither an early goal nor a soft option. Much preliminary work will need to be accomplished with the patient before the reins can be safely handed over – and alas, there can never at the outset be any guarantee of reaching such a stage. Some patients may prefer to hand over the control of their lives to health care workers precisely because they feel inadequate to assume full responsibility for how they conduct themselves, and often with good reason.

An important principle of behavioural re-education and medical care remains to be considered at this point. Alone and unaided in grappling with what may be seen as an intractable problem, the victim may capitulate or take flight; with social support, he or she may gain the strength to carry on struggling. Individual therapy has its place, always provided that the client is capable of a one-to-one relationship, but in the long run it is far from cost-effective. Moreover the social facilitation inherent in group therapy has an honourable history, as demonstrated by the success story of Alcoholics Anonymous and kindred organizations. Whereas alcoholism is not strictly a disease but (like other addictions) a maladaptive form of behaviour, the self-help movement has extended to many disorders to be found in standard medical textbooks. In the field of neurology, for example, these encompass rare diseases such as myasthenia gravis as well as the more common ones such as multiple sclerosis. They may cater for those predominantly affected in early life (e.g. head injury) or later life (e.g. stroke). If in some instances it is the patient's relatives who have most to gain from joining, no matter; either way a need is being met that may be hard to meet in any other way. Evidence as to the effectiveness of most of these self-help groups is missing or at best inconclusive, but they show no sign of waning in popularity. At all events this chapter will end with a brief account of what can be done to reinforce the individual efforts of the chronic back pain sufferer.

The case for organized self-help

The National Back Pain Association (NBPA), founded in 1968, is the only British organization that is devoted solely to caring for back pain sufferers. Its declared objectives are as follows:

1 To help prevent back pain by educating people in the correct use of their bodies.
2 To form local branches for disseminating advice and information.
3 To raise funds for research into the causes and treatment of back pain.

Currently it has upwards of 3,500 members and nearly 50 branches spread widely (but not evenly) throughout the country. It is administered by a small headquarters staff at Teddington, Middlesex, with the support of six regional directors. Research based in hospitals and university departments has attracted funds of approximately £150,000, and embraces both mechanical and social/psychological aspects. The association publishes a number of helpful leaflets and manuals on back pain and its prevention as well as a quarterly magazine (*TalkBack*). Anyone wishing to contact the association should address correspondence to NBPA, Grundy House, 31–33 Park Road, Teddington, Middlesex TW11 0AB, or telephone 01–977 5474.

Little appears to be known about the characteristics of those who join any kind of self-help group, which must vary with the nature of the group. It might be predicted that only those with a positive attitude to helping themselves would be drawn towards them; yet despite a nucleus of devotees there is often a brisk turnover in membership which suggests that rapid disenchantment may be a prime hazard. Monthly meetings with invited speakers from a wide range of disciplines have become the normal pattern for branches of the NBPA, followed by refreshments and ample time for discussion. This does of course entail a risk of confusion from a multiplicity of viewpoints, or enhancement of the impulse to 'shop around' for that elusive magic remedy. My own personal appearances have provoked only one member of the audience into attending our weekly clinic, and she shows promise of becoming one of our major success stories after an invigorating spell at the Wolfson Centre (p. 64). However, we could do with a lot more information about those who join and the consequences of so doing, whether purely subjective or reliably measurable. For if recognition of the need for self-help is truly a prerequisite of learning to cope with an otherwise intractable problem, then health care workers could presumably be more active in urging their chronic patients to become members of the association. Although non-joiners abound in all walks of life, it seems a pity that potential members should be prevented from joining by ignorance of its existence.

As a modest step towards collecting relevant data, I analysed a more or less consecutive series of fifty letters received by the association over the previous few months. These were pleas for help from sufferers or their relatives, and were answered in longhand by the association's scientific advisor, Dr S. K. Manstead. Those who write to Headquarters are unlikely to be members, otherwise they would be in contact with their local branch, yet they are possible recruits. Correspondents were of all ages (though age was not always given) and from all points of the compass, with the Home Counties predominating. Some lived alone, others mentioned the adverse effects of their disability on a partner. All were clearly desperate and some felt abandoned by doctors, having run the gamut of diverse remedial measures from physiotherapy to surgery. Associated disabilities ranged from amputation to blindness. A young mother confessed to a fear of spinal cancer such that she found herself weeping at her son's school concert in case she would not live until the next Christmas – her letter began 'It's your doomy friend again'.

A notable feature of this small series was the preponderance of women, as already remarked of hospital out-patients referred for psychological evaluation. This evidently also applies to telephone callers (Manstead, personal communication). Women are known for their more highly developed tactile sense, which could be taken to imply a lower pain threshold; it is also generally agreed that they have lower pain tolerance (Woodrow *et al*. 1972), which in laboratory studies might be partly a function of their more socially acceptable readiness to call a halt to painful stimulation. Although women may find it easier to express their anguish, be it verbally or in writing, and are on the whole less likely to be taken to task by society for unabashed self-disclosure, this is no warrant for inferring that men are more stoical by nature. A fair proportion of our more grievously distressed clinic patients have been male.

Since GPs are normally the first port of call for the acute back pain sufferer and will remain in touch at the chronic stage if only for repeat prescriptions, there is a good case for displaying the association's basic information leaflet in their surgeries, especially within a ten-mile radius of local branches. There would then need to be a brief monitoring exercise (say over a span of six months) to measure the effect on recruitment of new members, for which the association would have to be responsible. A major obstacle is the reduced mobility of many sufferers, who would be reluctant to travel if it meant more than a 20–30-minute journey by car (corresponding to something like ten miles in an urban area). Patients have a right to complain if supposedly therapeutic measures have the unfortunate effect of rendering them even more handicapped in the short term. This is why offers of a domiciliary visit from health care workers are usually so welcome; and much as one might want to argue that new incentives for getting out and about are in themselves therapeutic, this is not the sort of argument to appeal to those who have yet to be convinced of the merits of self-help.

What matters ultimately is that facilities for the social promotion of self-help should be widely publicized, so that the individual can be in a position to choose between the camaraderie of fellow sufferers or self-imposed but far from splendid isolation. Not uncommonly it is of some benefit also to discover from direct observation that others can be much worse afflicted than oneself, as happens every time a pain patient is admitted to the Wolfson Centre. Pain can be crippling, but surely less so than severe hemiplegia following a stroke. The opportunity to meet fellow sufferers in a controlled environment, and exposure to a wealth of professional experience in the management of chronic pain, are not to be dismissed lightly.

Regular discussion groups, professionally led but not dominated by experts, have been a feature of some multidisciplinary pain programmes in the USA (e.g. Sternbach 1974). A thoughtful study by Linssen and Zitman (1984) took account of patients' own comments at the end of a preliminary exercise in planning a more effective sequel. Group experience can be put to good use, not only in confronting individual members with their self-defeating or manipulative tendencies (since others are not easily fooled), but in encouraging all members to learn from one another. For in the end it is patients who have most to teach about the nature of human suffering, individually or collectively.

Chapter seven

Epilogue

In launching into a treatise on chronic back pain we have rightly or wrongly postponed any attempt to consider the quality of pain as a more general phenomenon. The opening chapter was restricted to the medical aspects of our subject; and whilst subsequent chapters have made passing mention of other forms of pain, these have not been allowed to intrude more than momentarily. In a sense the review has been tied to a rather narrow perspective by my own clinical experience, which has been largely confined to pain of musculoskeletal origin. But before concluding we ought to bear in mind that clinical pain may be either more localized or more diffuse than the syndromes under discussion.

A medical journalist, reviewing a new book about the knee in the context of sports injuries (*Daily Telegraph*, 29 March 1988), pointed out that 'Not only housemaids suffer knee trouble, virtually all of us have a problem at some time in this vulnerable joint'. Perhaps so, yet it would be hard to envisage a psychological monograph on the painful knee, the effects of which are presumably less far-reaching than those of the painful back. In contrast, the pain of a more pervasive disorder such as rheumatoid arthritis is quite likely to spread diffusely through every aspect of daily living, thereby causing even more distress than chronic back pain if that were possible. So we must not lose sight of the infinite variety of pain experience, not only within any one disorder but also between different sites and pathologies.

What, then, can be said about the nature and quality of pain from a more general standpoint? When discussing the varieties of pain experience Melzack and Wall begin with an obvious point but one that may none the less bear repetition:

> Because pain is a private, personal experience, it is impossible
> for us to know precisely what someone else's pain feels like.
> No man can possibly know what it is like to have menstrual
> cramps or labour pain. Nor can the psychologically healthy
> person know what a psychotic patient is feeling when he says
> he has excruciating pain.
>
> (Melzack and Wall 1988: 41)

It was with a view to eliciting the major properties of pain experience that Melzack (1975) devised the McGill Pain Questionnaire,
which seeks to delineate the sensory, affective, and evaluative[1]
components through a distinctive constellation of words. Sufferers
from diverse types of pain (e.g. menstrual, dental, neuralgic,
metastatic) tended to endorse a characteristic set of verbal descrip-
tors for each. Thus the test was potentially useful as a diagnostic
instrument, and was applied to back pain sufferers by Prieto *et
al.* (1980). This method of tapping pain experience has not been
universally accepted, but it does at least demonstrate that – for all
its essentially private nature – pain is also a form of interpersonal
communication. To rely exclusively on language for this purpose
would be unsatisfactory, since not all of us are equally skilful
with words; and anyone observing the social interaction of pain
sufferers would soon become aware of an array of *non-verbal*
signals which tell their own story. Clearly those of us who work
with pain patients must not only listen carefully to what they have
to say, but even more assiduously take note of what they do not
say. Much of what they may be trying to convey will be by gesture,
facial expression, tone of voice, or other coded message. The level
of overt complaint may be muted or vociferous; it is often the
obbligato accompaniment that tells us what we really need to
know. The communicative function of pain is what makes it so
powerful in the sphere of marital and other close relationships.
This is not to deny that the desert island castaway would be
capable of *feeling* pain, although he (or she) might well be somewhat discouraged by the lack of an audience.

Pain experience and pain expression are influenced by a number
of different factors. The lesser impact of injury sustained in battle
as compared with surgical wounds of the same severity inflicted
upon civilians has been immortalized by Beecher (1959: 165), who
found that there was

> no simple direct relationship between the wound per se and

the pain experienced. The pain is in very large part determined by other factors, and of great importance here is the significance of the wound . . . in the wounded soldier [the response to injury] was relief, thankfulness at his escape alive from the battlefield, even euphoria; to the civilian his major surgery was a depressing, calamitous event.

This is no more than a dramatic illustration of what has since become a commonplace finding, namely that the meaning of pain is heavily dependent on its context. Past experience contributes to the extent that, as a result of family and other environmental influences, the individual may have become either sensitized or hardened to pain. Cultural factors have also been implicated by some authorities, notably Zborowski (1952), whose classic observation that Italian and Jewish patients were more vocal in pain display than Old American and Irish patients seems to have gone unchallenged (indeed, it has been reinforced by psychophysiological experiments, e.g. Sternbach and Tursky 1965). The cognitive therapy movement should serve to highlight the social aspects of pain; and just as Davidson (1976) in the context of therapeutic compliance has pleaded for a closer liaison between clinicians and social scientists, so in pain management we may hope for a more fruitful collaboration between those who treat and those who merely take the world apart.

Towards a better service for pain patients

Clinical and experimental work over the past two decades especially may have helped to promote conceptual clarity, yet it is still uncertain how far this is reflected in improved services to patients. Two firm priorities have emerged from recent research, including work in progress. First, we need to find methods of discriminating more sharply between pain as such and the distress to which it gives rise – or which in some cases may have been its primary source. Clinical psychologists, we suggest, have so far been more active in developing their practical skills as agents of behavioural change than in applying their theoretical knowledge to the analysis of human distress. And it may be that the latter needs to be understood and as far as possible alleviated before tangible benefits can be expected.

Second, we must pay more attention to stressful life events in their capacity for reducing pain tolerance. For even if pain *threshold* – the level of stimulation at which pain is registered – varies between individuals, it is the greater variability of pain *tolerance* that is central to coping behaviour. As noted in an earlier chapter, despite innumerable studies of life events in relation to depression and other psychiatric disorders, there has been remarkably little interest in plotting their relationship to chronic pain. Had my foresight stretched to including a schedule of life events routinely in my interviews with pain patients, this monograph would almost certainly have benefited.

Stress may be either sharp and sudden, as with the woman whose daughter had just become dangerously addicted to heroin; or it may be constant and cumulative, as with the man whose teenage son had suffered from muscular dystrophy for most of his life and was considered unlikely to reach the age of 20. Either way it cannot readily be dissociated from the experience of pain, nor can the therapist afford to disregard it. The impact of life stress can be measured by asking the individual to record which of a standard series of events have occurred within the past year or two, at the same time indicating the degree of upset experienced on a scale of (say) 1–10. Cooper *et al.* (1988) have culled a forty-two-item schedule from the voluminous literature, embracing bereavement, illness in the family, marital problems, unemployment, and a variety of less obviously traumatic experiences. The shrewd clinician will make a point of enquiring into such matters when faced with any stress-related disorder, but without a formal questionnaire it is easy to miss vital information. It is not sufficient to know whether a particular event has occurred: it is equally if not more important to assess how the patient has reacted to it. Finally, the amount of support available from close associates has to be gauged as far as possible – no easy task under the conditions of a typical doctor's surgery or hospital out-patient clinic. Often enough it is only after a thorough appraisal of the patient's current life situation that one can hope to be in a position to devise a realistic plan of management. (This is not to dismiss the relevance of past history, yet it has taken many decades to set the psychoanalytic emphasis on early childhood in proper perspective.)

Cooper and his colleagues have also looked into the question of occupational stress, which appears to have been a major factor with some of our patients. Research has shown that two critical dimensions governing the level of stress in a job are *demand* and *control*, which refer to pressure of work and degree of individual autonomy respectively. Thus the most stressful occupations are those with relentless demands and little or no control over how they are to be met. Nurses, policemen, and prison officers come to mind as striking examples of those who work under a great deal of stress, and in our experience they are over-represented among back pain sufferers. For example, they accounted for no fewer than 10 of the 50 patients analysed in Chapter 4.

Of course, it will not do to pretend that social and occupational stress are crucial factors in any and every case of chronic back pain. Despite a preponderance of unknown causes, which Loeser (1980) has estimated at 70 per cent, it remains likely that mechanical causes are the most common even if they cannot always be identified, and treatment must be planned on this basis. However, most of the patients attending our weekly clinic have run the gamut of physicians, surgeons, physiotherapists, osteopaths, and chiropractors without gaining any semblance of control over their pain. Such persistent and at times almost compulsive searching for a cure has opened the way for others to explore the stresses with which the patient has had to contend; yet the case histories already quoted bear witness to an astonishing lack of interest in how he or she has coped or failed to cope with them. In the quest for a mechanical solution to what may have started as a mechanical problem, the owner of the bad back has almost vanished without trace.

It is hard to judge how many of these difficult patients could have been helped by more appropriate interventions earlier in their passage towards chronicity. Unhappily the National Health Service is not geared to the prompt introduction of new approaches, nor does the private sector enjoy much of an advantage in this respect. Doctors undoubtedly need to be better educated about the nature and management of chronic pain, whilst clinical psychologists are still a pathetically small workforce (about 1,500 at the time of writing). We do not know what the future may hold in store, but at this stage it would be foolish to underestimate the magnitude of the problem. Nor is the unashamedly aggressive stance of some American workers to be recommended. Tempting as it may sometimes be to seize on the use of pain as a weapon of interpersonal control (Szasz 1968; Sternbach 1974), a firm commitment to such an interpretation would soon become self-defeating and might well do more harm than good. Thus we cannot fully sympathize with Sternbach and Rusk when they write – albeit entertainingly – about 'alternatives to the pain career'. They may feel justified in challenging the patient's goals for living, but the cheerful brutality of the following excerpt might be unacceptable in an NHS clinic:

> When asked how they would live tomorrow if their pain were removed today, patients usually say they want to go back to work. This is automatic, as they have often been accused of trying to avoid work, and find it necessary to assert their honest intentions. We react incredulously: 'Work! what on earth for? That doesn't sound like much fun!' The patient then describes how difficult it is to make ends meet on his meager disability pension, how boring it is sitting around with nothing to do, etc.
>
> (Sternbach and Rusk 1973: 323)

This is an instance of what has come to be known as *paradoxical injunction*, which should be used sparingly even if it is worth trying when all else has failed. Shock tactics are not generally the most promising route to self-help.

Most health care workers beyond the first flush of youth will have suffered the odd episode of back pain, whereas few will have become chronically incapacitated by it. This means that, in order to have respect for the patient as a person, they will need to cultivate that triad of virtues made famous by Truax and Carkhuff (1967): empathy, genuineness, and non-possessive warmth. Not all good therapists can lay claim to all three of these in equal measure, and most bad therapists are deficient in one or more. But if there is any single quality that working with pain patients calls for above all else it must be empathy – one needs to be able to imagine what chronic suffering is like. Obviously any competent therapist should be able to transcend the limits of personal experience, for this is part of what professional training is designed to achieve. The person who has never experienced pain, anxiety, or depression is unlikely to be a mature adult, and ought certainly to steer clear of therapeutic practice. It is to be hoped that as the experience of chronic back pain becomes better understood, so its management will become more effective. Whatever the scope for prevention, it seems safe to assume that this dreadful scourge of *Homo erectus* will be with us for all time. Teaching people to cope with their pain, and in so doing to ward off its more demoralizing effects, is an extraordinary and everlasting challenge.

Appendix I

CONFIDENTIAL

THE ROBERT JONES AND AGNES HUNT ORTHOPAEDIC
HOSPITAL, OSWESTRY, SHROPSHIRE
Department for Spinal Disorders

Name .... Date ....

Address .... Age ....

.... DoB ....

Occupation .... Hospital No. ....

How long have you had back pain? ..... years ..... months ..... weeks

How long have you had leg pain? ..... years ..... months ..... weeks

Please read:

This questionnaire has been designed to give the doctor information as
to how your back pain has affected your ability to manage in everyday
life. Please answer every section, and mark in each section only the *ONE
BOX* which applies to you. We realise you may consider that two of the
statements in any one section relate to you, but please just *mark the box
which most clearly describes your problem.*

Section 1: PAIN INTENSITY

☐ I can tolerate the pain I have without having to use pain killers
☐ The pain is bad but I manage without taking pain killers
☐ Pain killers give complete relief from pain
☐ Pain killers give moderate relief from pain
☐ Pain killers give very little relief from pain
☐ Pain killers have no effect on the pain and I do not use them

Section 2: PERSONAL CARE (washing, dressing, etc.)

- ☐ I can look after myself normally without causing extra pain
- ☐ I can look after myself normally but it causes extra pain
- ☐ It is painful to look after myself and I am slow and careful
- ☐ I need some help but manage most of my personal care
- ☐ I need help every day in most aspects of self-care
- ☐ I do not get dressed, wash with difficulty and stay in bed

Section 3: LIFTING

- ☐ I can lift heavy weights without extra pain
- ☐ I can lift heavy weights but it gives me extra pain
- ☐ Pain prevents me from lifting heavy weights off the floor, but I can manage if they are conveniently positioned, e.g. on a table
- ☐ Pain prevents me from lifting heavy weights but I can manage light to medium weights if they are conveniently positioned
- ☐ I can only lift very light weights
- ☐ I cannot lift or carry anything at all

Section 4: WALKING

- ☐ Pain does not prevent me walking any distance
- ☐ Pain prevents me walking more than one mile
- ☐ Pain prevents me walking more than half a mile
- ☐ Pain prevents me walking more than a quarter of a mile
- ☐ I can only walk using a stick or crutches
- ☐ I am in bed most of the time and have to crawl to the toilet

Section 5: SITTING

- ☐ I can sit in any chair as long as I like
- ☐ I can only sit in my favourite chair as long as I like
- ☐ Pain prevents me from sitting more than one hour
- ☐ Pain prevents me from sitting more than half an hour
- ☐ Pain prevents me from sitting more than ten minutes
- ☐ Pain prevents me from sitting at all

Section 6: STANDING

- ☐ I can stand as long as I want without extra pain
- ☐ I can stand as long as I want but it gives me extra pain
- ☐ Pain prevents me from standing for more than one hour
- ☐ Pain prevents me from standing for more than half an hour
- ☐ Pain prevents me from standing for more than ten minutes
- ☐ Pain prevents me from standing at all

Section 7: SLEEPING

- ☐ Pain does not prevent me from sleeping well
- ☐ I can only sleep well using tablets
- ☐ With or without tablets I have less than six hours' sleep

☐ With or without tablets I have less than four hours' sleep
☐ With or without tablets I have less than two hours' sleep
☐ Pain prevents me from sleeping at all

Section 8: SEX LIFE

☐ My sex life is normal and causes no extra pain
☐ My sex life is normal but causes some extra pain
☐ My sex life is nearly normal but is very painful
☐ My sex life is severely restricted by pain
☐ My sex life is nearly absent because of pain
☐ Pain prevents any sex life at all

Section 9: SOCIAL LIFE

☐ My social life is normal and gives me no extra pain
☐ My social life is normal but increases the degree of pain
☐ Pain has no significant effect on my social life apart from limiting my more energetic interests (dancing, etc.)
☐ Pain has restricted my social life and I do not go out as often
☐ Pain has restricted my social life to my home
☐ I have no social life because of pain

Section 10: TRAVELLING

☐ I can travel anywhere without extra pain
☐ I can travel anywhere but it gives me extra pain
☐ Pain is bad but I manage journeys over two hours
☐ Pain restricts me to journeys of less than an hour
☐ Pain restricts me to short necessary journeys under 30 minutes
☐ Pain prevents me travelling except to the doctor or hospital

COMMENTS ....

Appendix II

(Mark 'X' against items that are not applicable)

Name_____

Age _____ Date _____

Occupation _____

Years of unemployment due to back pain _____

Duration of back pain_____

Number of back operations_____

Age of spouse _____

Occupation of spouse _____

No. of children (give sex and age) _____

Is your pain constantly present?_____

Does your pain vary:
by the minute/by the hour/by the day/by the week/by the month?

How many different specialists have you seen for your back pain?
Please write names and professions here:

111

In the *Pain* column, which you should complete first, please indicate how often you would engage in the various activities *even when your pain is at its worst*. In the *No pain* column, indicate how often you would expect to perform these activities if you were *free from pain*. Enter the appropriate number in each case, or mark an 'X' against any item which does not apply.

0	1	2	3
Never/seldom	Sometimes	Quite often	Very often

		Pain	No pain
1.	Go to parties or dances	....	....
2.	Go for pleasure rides in cars	....	....
3.	Go to pubs or wine bars	....	....
4.	Go to restaurants or cafés	....	....
5.	Go to social clubs (e.g. bingo, party political)	....	....
6.	Spend time on sports or games with others	....	....
7.	Have sexual intercourse	....	....
8.	Visit family or friends	....	....
9.	Go to the cinema or theatre	....	....
10.	Invite visitors to your home	....	....
11.	Do the cooking	....	....
12.	Go up and down stairs	....	....
13.	Do heavy gardening (e.g. digging a flower-bed)	....	....
14.	Do odd jobs around the house (e.g. painting a door)	....	....
15.	Do odd jobs outside the home (e.g. cleaning the car)	....	....
16.	Go shopping	....	....
17.	Do gentle housework (e.g. dusting)	....	....
18.	Do light gardening (e.g. pruning)	....	....
19.	Do heavy housework (e.g. hoovering, washing floors)	....	....
20.	Do a day's work outside the home	....	....

Notes

Chapter 1

1 There have been one or two promising leads in the more recent literature. For example, Murphy and Cornish (1984) reported correct classification of 41 out of 48 patients (85 per cent) who were seen initially at the acute stage. All but 4 of the 28 patients who became chronically affected had shown an early pattern of deep musculoskeletal rather than peripheral pain at numerous body sites, in a setting of high anxiety and low activity.

2 What this author fails to consider in this summary account (but see also Porter 1986) is the regrettable ease with which stress can be applied to the spine. It is not merely a question of poor posture, faulty lifting techniques and so on, but of having to adapt to a working environment designed with scant regard for even the average human frame. Housewives, for example, are under repeated daily stress from furniture and equipment ill-suited to their physical needs, whilst drivers of either sex have only recently begun to benefit from vehicle manufacturers' belated attention to the need for lumbar support when confined behind a wheel, sometimes for hours on end. What has come to be known as the *ergonomic* approach to the relief of back pain will be discussed towards the end of this chapter as well as later in the book.

3 Partial or complete severance of the spinal cord, arising from trauma more commonly than from disease and leading to paraplegia or tetraplegia, is of course a different matter. Here the most serious consequence is loss of mobility and sensation due to interference with the crucial nerve supply. Any experience of pain is apt to be overshadowed by intense feelings of helplessness.

Chapter 2

1 A one-armed tennis player (H. Redl of Austria) was astonishingly effective in the early post-war era of the Wimbledon doubles' championships.

2 Remarkable comebacks have been achieved by disabled athletes even after spinal surgery. To draw on tennis again, several top-class players

including at least one Wimbledon champion have defied all prediction by improving on their pre-operative level, outstanding though it had been.

3 Conversely, undue reliance on the ambulance or hospital car service is associated with magnified pain presentation.

Chapter 3

1 Alas, the story has an unhappy ending. On a visit to London, Fordyce was asked whether he was still in touch with the patient, to which he replied that she had died of a massive coronary about six years after the rehabilitation. Outwardly the husband seemed to have adapted to his loss, and he was clearly grateful for his wife's restoration to normal living for the last few years of her life, after almost twenty years of invalidism.

Chapter 4

1 Perfect consistency is not, of course, to be expected even over a short period from patients undergoing specialized rehabilitation, and indeed it would be a mark of insensitivity if no changes were recorded on any questionnaire items.

2 This patient was atypical in having originally approached me after my address to a local branch of the National Back Pain Association. She had received conflicting advice about surgery, and she then came to our clinic for the usual assessment. Instead of ending in theatre she spent three or four weeks at the Wolfson Centre and was duly impressed by the enthusiasm of the staff. During the follow-up period she no longer took to her bed for two or three days every month, preferring to soldier on as she had been taught.

3 Our own clinical judgement was clearly premature in this instance. When seen later, after a short spell at the Wolfson Centre, the patient had been retired from the Post Office on medical grounds and was not looking for other work. For the first time in the course of several meetings he seemed entirely relaxed and at peace with himself.

Chapter 5

1 Virtually equal numbers of men and women are referred to the clinic, but women predominate among patients seen for independent psychological assessment. The reason for this bias is not fully understood, but women may well be more adept at declaring their distress. For a full discussion of this complex issue, in the contrasted spheres of primary care and government employment respectively, see Briscoe (1982) and Jenkins (1985).

Chapter 7

1 There has been some controversy over whether the evaluative component of the McGill Pain Questionnaire is sufficiently distinct from the affective component, but a factorial study by Prieto *et al*. (1980) suggests that it is.

References

Ahern, D. K., Adams, A. E., and Follick, M. J. (1985) 'Emotional and marital disturbance in spouses of chronic low back pain patients', *Clinical Journal of Pain* 1: 69–74.

Alperson, B. L., Gottlieb, B., Hockersmith, V., and Koller, R. (1984) 'Self-management for medication reduction in a chronic back pain population', *IASP 4th World Congress, Seattle*.

Anderson, J. A. D. (1987) 'Back pain and occupation', in M. I. V. Jayson (ed.) *The Lumbar Spine and Back Pain* (3rd edn), Edinburgh: Churchill Livingstone.

Anderson, T. P., Cole, T. M., Gullickson, G., Hudgens, A., and Roberts, A. H. (1977) 'A treatment program by a multidisciplinary team', *Journal of Clinical Orthopedics* 129: 96–100.

Aronoff, G. M., Evans, W. O., and Kenders, P. L. (1983) 'A review of follow-up studies of multidisciplinary pain units', *Pain* 16: 1–11.

Barsky, A. J. (1981) 'Hidden reasons some patients visit doctors', *Annals of Internal Medicine* 94: 492–8.

Baxter, D. W. and Olszewski, J. (1960) 'Congenital insensitivity to pain', *Brain* 83: 381–93.

Beals, R. K. and Hickman, N. W. (1972) 'Industrial injuries of the back and extremities', *Journal of Bone and Joint Surgery* 54A (2): 1593–611.

Beecher, H. K. (1959) *Measurement of Subjective Responses*, New York: Oxford University Press.

Bernard, J. (1976) *The Future of Marriage*, Harmondsworth: Penguin.

Beyfus, D. (1968) *The English Marriage: What it is Like to be Married Today*, London: Weidenfeld & Nicolson.

Block, A. R. (1981) 'Investigation of the response of the spouse to chronic pain behaviour', *Psychosomatic Medicine* 43: 415–22.

Block, A. R. and Boyer, S. L. (1984) 'The spouse's adjustment to chronic pain: cognitive and emotional factors', *Social Science and Medicine* 19: 1313–17.

Block, A. R., Kremer, E. F., and Gaylor, M. (1980) 'Behavioral treatment of chronic pain: the spouse as a discriminative cue for pain behavior', *Pain* 9: 243–52.

Bokan, J. A., Reis, R. K., and Katon, W. J. (1981) 'Tertiary gain and chronic pain', *Pain* 10: 331–5.

Bond, M. R. (1984) *Pain: its Nature, Analysis and Treatment* (2nd edn), Edinburgh: Churchill Livingstone.

Briscoe, M. (1982) 'Sex differences in psychological well-being', *Psychological Medicine Monograph Supplement 1*, Cambridge: Cambridge University Press.

Broome, A. and Jellicoe, H. (1987) *Living with Pain: a Guide to Managing Pain*, Leicester: British Psychological Society/Methuen.

Connolly, R. C. (1982) 'Pain as a problem to the neurosurgeon', *Journal of the Royal Society of Medicine* 75: 160–5.

Cooper, C. L., Cooper, R. D., and Eaker, L. H. (1988) *Living with Stress*, Harmondsworth: Penguin.

Coughlan, A. K. and Humphrey, M. (1982) 'Presenile stroke: long-term outlook for patients and their families', *Rheumatology and Rehabilitation* 21: 115–22.

Craig, K. D. (1978) 'Social modeling influences on pain', in R. A. Sternbach (ed.) *The Psychology of Pain*, New York: Raven.

Crasilneck, H. B. (1979) 'Hypnosis in the control of chronic low back pain', *American Journal of Clinical Hypnosis* 22: 71–8.

Davidson, P. O. (1976) 'Therapeutic compliance', *Canadian Psychological Review* 17: 247–59.

Delvey, J. and Hopkins, L. (1982) 'Pain patients and their partners: the role of collusion in chronic pain', *Journal of Marriage and Marital Therapy* 7: 135–42.

DHSS (Department of Health and Social Security) (1979) *Report of the Working Group on Back Pain*, London: HMSO.

Derogatis, L. R. and Spencer, P. M. (1982) *The Brief Symptom Inventory (BSI): Administration, Scoring and Procedures Manual I*, Baltimore, Md.: Clinical Psychometrics Research.

Deyo, R. A. (1983) 'Conservative therapy for low back pain', *Journal of the American Medical Association* 250: 1052–62.

Deyo, R. A. and Diehl, A. K. (1986) 'Patient satisfaction with medical care for low back pain', *Spine* 11: 28–30.

Deyo, R. A., Diehl, A. K., and Rosenthal, M. (1986) 'How many days of bed rest for acute low back pain? A randomised clinical trial', *New England Journal of Medicine* 315: 1064–70.

Dillane, J. B., Fry, J., and Kalton, G. (1966) 'Acute back syndrome – a study from general practice', *British Medical Journal* ii: 82–4.

Dixon, A. St J. (1980) 'Diagnosis of low back pain: sorting the complainers', in M. I. V. Jayson (ed.) *The Lumbar Spine and Back Pain* (2nd edn), London: Pitman

Dixon, A. St J. (1987) Introduction to M. I. V. Jayson (ed.) *The Lumbar Spine and Back Pain* (3rd edn), Edinburgh: Churchill Livingstone.

Dunbar, J. (1980) 'Adhering to medical advice: a review', *International Journal of Mental Health* 9: 70–87.

Dunnell, K. and Cartwright, A. (1972) *Medicine Takers, Prescribers and Hoarders*, London: Routledge & Kegan Paul.

Edgar, M. A. (1984) 'Backache', *British Journal of Hospital Medicine* 32: 290–301.

Edwards, P. W., Zeichner, A., Kuczmierczyk, R., and Bocznowski, J. (1985) 'Familial pain models: the relationship between family history of pain and current pain experience', *Pain* 21: 379–84.

Fairbank, J. C. T., Cowper, J., Davies, J. B., and O'Brien, J. P. (1980) 'The Oswestry low back pain disability questionnaire', *Physiotherapy* 66 (8): 271–3.

Feuerstein, M., Sult, S., and Houle, M. (1985) 'Environmental stressors and chronic low back pain: life events, family and work environment', *Pain* 22: 295–307.

Fitzpatrick, R. M., Bury, M., Frank, A. O., and Donnelly, T. (1987) 'Problems in the assessment of outcome in a back pain clinic', *International Disability Studies* 9: 161–5.

Flor, H., and Turk, D. C. (1984) 'Etiological theories and treatment for chronic back pain: I. Somatic models and interventions', *Pain* 19: 105–21.

Flor, H., Haag, G., Turk, D. C., and Koehler, H. (1983) 'Efficacy of EMG biofeedback, pseudotherapy and conventional medical treatment for chronic rheumatic back pain', *Pain* 17: 21–31.

Flor, H., Kerns, R. D., and Turk, D. C. (1987) 'The role of spouse reinforcement, perceived pain, and activity levels of chronic pain patients', *Journal of Psychosomatic Research* 31: 251–9.

Flor, H., Turk, D. C., and Rudy, T. E. (1987) 'Pain and families. II: Assessment and treatment', *Pain* 30: 29–45.

Flor, H., Turk, D. C., and Scholz, O. B. (1987) 'Impact of chronic pain on the spouse: marital, emotional and physical consequences', *Journal of Psychosomatic Research* 31: 63–71.

Folkard, S., Glynn, C. J., and Lloyd, J. W. (1976) 'Diurnal variations and individual differences in the perception of intractable pain', *Journal of Psychosomatic Research* 20: 289–301.

Fordyce, W. E. (1976) *Behavioral Methods in Chronic Pain and Illness*, St Louis, Miss.: Mosby.

Fordyce, W. E., Brena, S. F., Holcomb, R. J., De Lateur, B. J., and Loeser, J. D. (1978) 'Relationship of patient semantic pain descriptions to physician diagnostic judgements, activity level measures and MMPI', *Pain* 5: 293–303.

Fordyce, W. E., Fowler, R. S., and De Lateur, B. (1968) 'An application of behavior modification technique to a problem of chronic pain', *Behaviour Research and Therapy* 6: 105–7.

Gentry, W. D., Shows, W. D., and Thomas, M. (1974) 'Chronic low back pain: a psychological profile', *Psychosomatics* 15: 174–7.

Gillmore, M. R. and Hill, C. T. (1981) 'Reactions to patients who complain of pain: effects of ambiguous diagnosis', *Journal of Applied Social Psychology* 11: 14–22.

Glass, J. B. (1979) 'Acute lumbar strain: clinical signs and prognosis', *Practitioner* 222: 821–5.

Hamblen, D. L. (1980) 'The role of surgery in low back pain', *Clinics in Rheumatic Diseases* 6: 191–216.

Hay, K. M. and Madders, J. (1971) 'Migraine treated by relaxation therapy', *Journal of the Royal College of General Practitioners* 21: 664–9.

Heinrich, R. L., Cohen, M. J., Nabiloff, B. D., Collins, G. A., and Bonebakker, A. D. (1985) 'Comparing physical and behaviour therapy for chronic low back pain on physical abilities, psychological distress and patients' perception', *Journal of Behavioural Medicine* 8: 61–78.

Higham, C., Ashcroft, C., and Jayson, M. I. V. (1983) 'Non-prescribed treatments in rheumatic diseases', *Practitioner* 227: 1201–5.

Hilgard, E. R. and Hilgard, J. (1986) *Hypnosis in the Relief of Pain* (2nd edn), Los Altos, Cal.: Kaufmann.

Hughes, A. M., Medley, I., Turner, G. N., and Bond, M. R. (1987) 'Psychogenic pain: a study of marital adjustment', *Acta Psychiatrica Scandinavica* 75: 166–70.

Humphrey, M. (1980) 'The problem of low back pain', in S. J. Rachman (ed.) *Contributions to Medical Psychology*, vol. 2, Oxford: Pergamon.

Humphrey, M. (1985) 'The role of the spouse in pain management', in E. Karas (ed.) *Current Issues in Clinical Psychology*, vol. 2, New York: Plenum.

Humphrey, M. and Jenkins, D. (1982) 'Personality factors in the rehabilitation of back pain sufferers', unpublished manuscript.

Humphrey, M. and Jones, N. (1987) 'Chronic pain and marital stability', *Stress Medicine* 3: 261–2.

Humphrey, M. and McNally, C. (1983) 'A scale for measuring pain avoidance', unpublished.

Ingham, J. G. and Miller, P. McC. (1979) 'Symptom prevalence and severity in a general practice population', *Journal of Epidemiology and Community Health* 33: 191–8.

Jayson, M. I. V. (1984) 'Difficult diagnoses in back pain', *British Medical Journal* 288: 740–1.

Jayson, M. I. V. (1987) *Back Pain: the Facts* (2nd edn), Oxford: Oxford University Press.

Jayson, M. I. V., Keegan, A., Million, R., and Tomlinson, I. (1984) 'A fibrinolytic defect in chronic back pain syndromes', *Lancet* ii: 1186–7.

Jenkins, R. (1985) 'Sex differences in minor psychiatric morbidity', *Psychological Medicine Monograph, Supplement 7*, Cambridge: Cambridge University Press.

Jones, B. N. H. (1985) 'Pain experience and activity level: a study of spinal patients undergoing rehabilitation', unpublished M.Sc. thesis, University of Surrey.

Karasu, T. B. (1979) 'Psychotherapy of the medically ill', *American Journal of Psychiatry* 136: 1–11.

Keefe, F. J., Block, A. R., Williams, R. B., and Surwit, R. S. (1981) 'Behavioural treatment of chronic low back pain: clinical outcome and individual differences in pain relief', *Pain* 11: 221–31.

Kreitman, N., Sainsbury, P., Pearce, K., and Costain, W. R. (1965) 'Hypochondriasis and depression in outpatients at a general hospital', *British Journal of Psychiatry* 111: 607–15.

Large, R. G. (1985) 'Prediction of treatment response in pain patients:

the illness self-concept repertory grid and EMG feedback', *Pain* 21: 279–87.

Lawrence, J. (1977) *Rheumatism in Populations*, London: Heinemann.

Ley, P. (1982) 'Satisfaction, compliance and communication', *British Journal of Clinical Psychology* 21: 241–54.

Linssen, A. C. G. and Zitman, F. G. (1984) 'Patient evaluation of a cognitive behavioural group programme for patients with low back pain', *Social Science & Medicine* 19: 1361–5.

Linton, S. J. (1985) 'The relationship between activity and chronic back pain', *Pain* 21: 289–94.

Litman, T. J. (1974) 'The family as the basic unit in health and medical care: a social behavioral overview', *Social Science & Medicine* 8: 495–9.

Litman, T. J. and Venters, M. (1979) 'Research on health care and the family: a methodological overview', *Social Science & Medicine* 13A: 379–85.

Loeser, J. D. (1980) 'Low back pain', in J. J. Bonica (ed.) *Pain*, New York: Raven.

McCauley, J. D., Thelen, M. H., Frank, R. G., Willard, R. R., and Callen, K. E. (1983) 'Hypnosis compared to relaxation in the outpatient management of chronic low back pain', *Archives of Physical Medicine and Rehabilitation* 64: 548–52.

MacDonald, E. B. (1984) 'Back pain, the risk factors and its prediction in work people', in J. Brothwood (ed.) *Occupational Aspects of Back Disorders*, London: Society of Occupational Medicine.

Magora, A. (1973) 'Investigation of the relationship between low back pain and occupation: 2. Psychological aspects', *Scandinavian Journal of Rehabilitation Medicine* 5: 191–6.

Main, C. J. (1987) 'Psychological approaches to management and treatment', in M. I. V. Jayson (ed.) *The Lumbar Spine and Back Pain* (3rd edn), Edinburgh: Churchill Livingstone.

Maruta, T. and Osborne, D. (1978) 'Sexual activity in chronic pain patients', *Psychosomatics* 19: 531–7.

Maruta, T., Osborne, D., Swanson, D. W., and Hallwig, J. M. (1981) 'Chronic pain patients and spouses: marital and sexual adjustment', *Mayo Clinic Proceedings* 56: 307–10.

Maruta, T., Swanson, D., and Swenson, W. M. (1976) 'Low back pain patients in a psychiatric population', *Mayo Clinic Proceedings* 51: 57–61.

Mellin, G., Järvikoski, A., and Verkasalo, M. (1984) 'Treatment of patients with chronic low back pain: comparison between rehabilitation centre and outpatient care', *Scandinavian Journal of Rehabilitation Medicine* 16: 77–84.

Melzack, R. (1975) 'The McGill Pain Questionnaire: major properties and scoring methods', *Pain* 1: 357–73.

Melzack, R. and Wall, P. D. (1988) *The Challenge of Pain* (2nd edn), Harmondsworth: Penguin.

Menges, L. J. (1981) 'Chronic pain patients: some psychological aspects', in S. Lipton and J. Miles (eds) *Persistent Pain*, vol. 3, London: Academic Press.

Merskey, H. and Spear, F. G. (1967) *Pain: Psychological and Psychiatric Aspects*, London: Baillière, Tindall & Cox.

Minuchin, S. (1974) *Families and Family Therapy*, Cambridge, Mass.: Harvard University Press.

Moore, J., Phipps, K., Marcer, D., and Lewith, G. (1985) 'Why do people seek treatment by alternative medicine?' *British Medical Journal* 290: 28–9.

Morrell, D. C. and Wale, C. J. (1976) 'Symptoms perceived and recorded by patients', *Journal of the Royal College of General Practitioners* 26: 398–403.

Murphy, K. A. and Cornish, R. D. (1984) 'Prediction of chronicity in acute low back pain', *Archives of Physical Medicine and Rehabilitation* 65: 334–7.

Nagi, S. Z., Burk, R. D., and Potter, H. R. (1965) 'Back disorders and rehabilitation achievement', *Journal of Chronic Diseases* 18: 181–97.

Nagi, S. Z., Riley, L. E., and Newby, L. G. (1973) 'A social epidemiology of back pain in a general population', *Journal of Chronic Diseases* 26: 769–79.

Nelson, M. A. (1987) 'Indications for spinal surgery in low back pain', in M. I. V. Jayson (ed.) *The Lumbar Spine and Back Pain* (3rd edn), Edinburgh: Churchill Livingstone.

Painter, J. R., Seres, J. L., and Newman, R. I. (1980) 'Assessing benefits of the pain center: why some patients regress', *Pain* 8: 101–13.

Payne, B. and Norfleet, M. A. (1986) 'Chronic pain and the family: a review', *Pain* 26: 1–22.

Pilowsky, I., Chapman, C. R., and Bonica, J. J. (1977) 'Pain, depression and illness behaviour in a pain clinic population', *Pain* 4: 183–92.

Pilowsky, I. and Spence, N. D. (1975) 'Patterns of illness behaviour in patients with intractable pain', *Journal of Psychosomatic Research* 19: 279–87.

Pilowsky, I. and Spence, N. D. (1976) 'Is illness behaviour related to chronicity in patients with intractable pain?' *Pain* 2: 167–73.

Porter, R. W. (1983) *Understanding Back Pain* (Patient Handbook 13), Edinburgh: Churchill Livingstone.

Porter, R. W. (1986) *Management of Back Pain*, Edinburgh: Churchill Livingstone.

Price, D. D., McGrath, P. A., Rafii, A., and Buckingham, B. (1983) 'The validation of visual analogue scales as ratio scale measures for chronic and experimental pain', *Pain* 17: 45–56.

Prieto, E. J., Hopson, L., Bradley, L. A., Byrne, M., Geisinger, K. F., Midax, D., and Marchisello, P. J. (1980) 'The language of low back pain: factor structure of the McGill Pain Questionnaire', *Pain* 8: 11–19.

Reilly, D. T. (1983) 'Young doctors' views on alternative medicine', *British Medical Journal* 287: 337–9.

Richards, J. S., Meredith, R. L., Nepomuceno, C., Fine, P. R., and Bennett, G. (1980) 'Psychosocial aspects of chronic pain in spinal cord injury', *Pain* 8: 355–66.

Ridgeway, V. and Mathews, A. (1982) 'Psychological preparation for surgery: a comparison of methods', *British Journal of Clinical Psychology* 21: 271–80.

Roberts, A. H. and Reinhardt, L. (1980) 'The behavioral management of chronic pain: long-term follow-up with comparison groups', *Pain* 8: 151–62.

Rose, H. J. (1975) 'The lives of patients before presentation with pain in the neck or back', *Journal of the Royal College of General Practitioners* 25: 771–2.

Rosenstiel, A. K. and Keefe, F. J. (1983) 'The use of coping strategies in chronic low back pain patients: relationship to patient characteristics and current adjustment', *Pain* 17: 33–44.

Rowat, K. M. and Knafl, K. A. (1985) 'Living with chronic pain: the spouse's perspective', *Pain* 23: 259–71.

Roy, R. (1982) 'Marital and family issues in patients with chronic pain: a review', *Psychotherapy and Psychosomatics* 37: 1–12.

RCGP (Royal College of General Practitioners) (1979) *Morbidity Statistics from General Practice 1971–1972. Second National Study* (Studies on Medical and Population Subjects, no. 36), London: HMSO.

Ryle, A. (1966) 'A marital patterns test for use in psychiatric research', *British Journal of Psychiatry* 112: 285–93.

Sanders, S. H. (1983) 'Component analysis of a behavioral treatment program for chronic low-back pain', *Behavior Therapy* 14: 697–705.

Satir, V. (1967) *Conjoint Family Therapy*, 1st edn, Palo Alto, Cal.: Science and Behavior Books.

Scott, J. and Huskisson, E. C. (1976) 'Graphic representation of pain', *Pain* 2: 175–84.

Seligman, M. (1975) *Helplessness. On Depression, Development, and Death*, San Francisco: W. H. Freeman.

Sifneos, P. E. (1973) 'Is dynamic psychotherapy contraindicated in a large number of patients with psychosomatic diseases?' *Psychotherapy and Psychosomatics* 21: 133–6.

Silver, B. V. and Blanchard, E. G. (1978) 'Biofeedback and relaxation training in the treatment of psychophysiological disorders: or, are the machines really necessary?' *Journal of Behavioural Medicine* 1: 217–39.

Silverman, L. (1977) 'Low back pain: a review of the psychological literature', unpublished manuscript, Oxford Rehabilitation Research Unit.

Simpson, G. (1984) 'Ergonomic problems and solutions', in J. Brothwood (ed.) *Occupational Aspects of Back Disorders*, London: Society of Occupational Medicine.

Skevington, S. M. (1983a) 'Activities as indices of illness behaviour in chronic pain', *Pain* 15: 295–307.

Skevington, S. M. (1983b) 'Chronic pain and depression: universal or personal helplessness?' *Pain* 15: 309–17.

Spanier, G. B. (1976) 'Measuring dyadic adjustment: new scales for assessing the quality of marriage and similar dyads', *Journal of Marriage and the Family* 38: 15–28.

Spielberger, R. A., Gorsuch, R. L., and Lushene, R. E. (1970) *Manual for the State-Trait Anxiety Inventory*, Palo Alto, Cal.: Consulting Psychologists Press.

Sternbach, R. A. (1963) 'Congenital insensitivity to pain: a review', *Psychological Bulletin* 60: 252–64.

Sternbach, R. A. (1974) *Pain Patients: Traits and Treatment*, New York: Academic Press.

Sternbach, R. A. and Rusk, T. N. (1973) 'Alternatives to the pain career', *Psychotherapy: Theory, Research and Practice* 10: 321–4.

Sternbach, R. A. and Tursky, B. (1965) 'Ethnic differences among housewives in psychophysical and skin potential responses to electric shock', *Psychophysiology* 1: 241–6.

Stubbs, D. A., Buckle, P. W., Hudson, M. P., and Rivers, P. M. (1983) 'Back pain in the nursing profession: II. The effectiveness of training', *Ergonomics* 26: 767–79.

Stubbs, D. A. and Nicholson, A. S. (1979) 'Manual handling and back injuries in the construction industry: an investigation', *Journal of Occupational Accidents* 2: 179–90.

Swanson, D. W. and Maruta, T. (1980) 'The family's viewpoint of chronic pain', *Pain* 8: 163–6.

Swanson, D. W., Maruta, T., and Swenson, W. M. (1979) 'Results of behavior modification in the treatment of chronic pain', *Psychosomatic Medicine* 41: 55–61.

Swanson, D. W., Swenson, W. M., Maruta, T., and McPhee, M. C. (1976) 'Program for managing chronic pain', *Mayo Clinic Proceedings*, 51: 401–8.

Szasz, T. S. (1968) 'The psychology of persistent pain: a portrait of l'homme douloureux', in A. Soulairas, J. Cahn, and J. Charpentier (eds) *Pain*, New York: Academic Press.

Tan, S.-Y. (1982) 'Cognitive and cognitive-behavioural methods for pain control: a selective review', *Pain* 12: 201–28.

Tasto, D. L. and Hinkle, J. E. (1973) 'Muscle relaxation treatment for tension headaches', *Behaviour Research and Therapy* 11: 347–9.

Thomas, M., Grant, N., Marshall, J., and Stevens, J. (1983) 'Surgical treatment of low backache and sciatica', *Lancet* ii: 1437–9.

Thoreau, H. D. (1854) *Walden, or Life in the Woods*. Reissued in Penguin American Library (1983). Harmondsworth: Penguin.

Truax, C. B. and Carkhuff, R. R. (1967) *Toward Effective Counselling and Psychotherapy*, Chicago: Aldine.

Turk, D. C. and Flor, H. (1984) 'Etiological theories and treatments for chronic back pain: II Psychological models and interventions', *Pain* 19: 209–33.

Turk, D. C., Flor, H., and Rudy, T. E. (1987) 'Pain and families. I: Etiology, maintenance and psychosocial impact, *Pain* 30: 3–27.

Turk, D. C., Meichenbaum, D. H., and Berman, W. H. (1979) 'Application of biofeedback in the regulation of pain: a critical review', *Psychological Bulletin* 86: 1322–38.

Turk, D. C., Meichenbaum, D., and Genest, M. (1983) *Pain and Behavioral Medicine: a Cognitive-behavioral Perspective*, New York: Guilford.

Turner, J. A. (1982) 'Comparison of group progressive relaxation training and cognitive-behavioural group therapy for chronic low back pain', *Journal of Consulting and Clinical Psychology* 50: 757–65.

Turner, J. A. and Chapman, C. R. (1982a) 'Psychological interventions for chronic pain: a critical review. 1. Relaxation training and biofeedback', *Pain*, 12: 1–21.

Turner, J. A. and Chapman, C. R. (1982b) 'Psychological interventions for chronic pain: a critical review. 2. Operant conditioning, hypnosis and cognitive-behavioural therapy', *Pain* 12: 23–46.

Vincent, P. (1971) 'Factors influencing patient non-compliance: a theoretical approach', *Nursing Research* 20: 509–16.

Violon, A. and Giurgea, D. (1984) 'Familial models for chronic pain', *Pain* 18: 199–203.

Waddell, G. (1987) 'Understanding the patient with backache', in M. I. V. Jayson (ed.) *The Lumbar Spine and Back Pain* (3rd edn), Edinburgh: Churchill Livingstone.

Waddell, G., Bircher, M., Finlayson, D., and Main, C. J. (1984) 'Symptoms and signs: physical disease or illness behaviour?' *British Medical Journal* 289: 739–41.

Waddell, G., McCulloch, J. A., Kummel, E. G., and Venner, R. M. (1980) 'Non-organic physical signs in low back pain', *Spine* 5: 117–25.

Waddell, G., Main, C. J., Morris, M. W., Paola, M. di, and Gray, I. C. M. (1984) 'Chronic low back pain, psychologic distress and illness behaviour', *Spine* 9: 209–13.

Wallace, L. (1984) 'Psychological preparation for gynaecological surgery', in A. Broome and L. Wallace (eds) *Psychology and Gynaecological Problems*, London: Tavistock.

Waring, E. M. (1977) 'The role of the family in symptom selection and perpetuation in psychosomatic illness', *Psychotherapy and Psychosomatics* 28: 253–9.

Waring, E. M. (1982) 'Conjoint and marital therapy', in R. Roy and E. Tunks (eds) *Chronic Pain: Psychosocial Factors in Rehabilitation*, Baltimore, Md.: Williams & Wilkins.

Wells, N. (1985) *Back Pain*, London: Office of Health Economics.

Wharton, R. N., Yang, J. C., and Clark, W. C. (1984) 'Psychological distress and outcome of treatment for chronic pain patients', *IASP 4th World Congress, Seattle*.

White, A. W. M. (1966) 'The compensation back', *Applied Therapy* 8: 871–4.

Wiltse, L. L. and Rocchio, P. D. (1975) 'Pre-operative psychological tests as predictors of success of chemonucleolysis in the treatment of the low back syndrome', *Journal of Bone and Joint Surgery* 57A: 478–83.

Wood, P. H. N. (1980) 'Understanding back pain', in M. I. V. Jayson (ed.) *The Lumbar Spine and Back Pain* (2nd edn), London: Pitman.

Wood, P. H. N. and Badley, E. M. (1980) 'Epidemiology of back pain', in M. I. V. Jayson (ed.) *The Lumbar Spine and Back Pain* (2nd edn), London: Pitman.

Woodrow, K. M., Friedman, G. D., Siegelaub, A. B., and Collen, M.

F. (1972) 'Pain tolerance: differences according to age, sex and race', *Psychosomatic Medicine* 34: 548–56.

Zborowski, M. (1952) 'Cultural components in responses to pain', *Journal of Social Issues* 8: 16–30.

Index

Abingdon Pain Relief Clinic 53
abscesses 9
accidents *see* injuries
activity: level of 50–68, 74, 81, 89, 93
acupuncture 12, 14
adaptability: teaching in 77
aetiology 6–10; accidents 20–1, 22–3, 24, 43–4; degenerative changes 8, 10, 29; inflammatory conditions 7, 10, 17–18; intervertebral disc displacement 5–6, 8, 10, 13; mechanical causes 7, 8, 13, 105; psychogenic causes 7–8, 33, 46; traumatic causes 9, 10
after-care 39
age of patients 20–1, 22, 33, 41, 85
Ahern, D. K. 38
alienation 31
Alperson, B. L. 78
alternative medicine 14–15, 87; *see also* individual techniques
anaesthetics 12
analgesics 12
Anderson, J. A. D. 22
Anderson, T. P. 73
ankylosing spondylitis 52
antidepressive medication 67
anti-inflammatory agents 12
Aronoff, G. M. 82
arthritis 21; *see also* rheumatoid arthritis
assertion training 74

attribution theory 66
audiovisual aids 79
autogenic relaxation training 74
avoidance of pain 50–68, 89, 93

back pain: interdisciplinary approach to 2, 69, 81–3, 100; medical aspects of 1–16; multidisciplinary working group on 10; purpose of 2–3; social and industrial results of 10–11, 15; spontaneous remission of 3, 13, 82; symptomatic nature of 6, 10–12; treatment of 12–13
Badley, E. M. 11
Barsky, A. J. 90
Baxter, D. W. 2
Beals, R. K. 19
bed rest 3, 10, 12, 39, 87
Beecher, H. K. 102
behaviour therapy 79
behavioural concepts: application to study of chronic pain 37–41, 51–3, 67, 71, 73, 74, 75
behavioural re-education 38–9, 40, 51, 67, 71, 73, 74, 96
behavioural sciences 90
bereavement 21, 104
Berman, W. H. 77
Bernard, J. 21
Beyfus, D. 32
biofeedback 71, 74, 76–7
Bircher, M. 2, 69, 72
Blanchard, E. G. 76